What the Mind Sees, the Body Feels, Creates and Attracts

LEAH MARMULLA

Copyright ©2019 Leah Marmulla

ISBN-10 164550283X
ISBN-13 9781645502838

All rights reserved. No part of this book may be reproduced, scanned, or distributed in any printed or electronic form without permission.

I have just finished reading Leah's book What the Mind Sees, Feels, Creates and Attracts-I am so pleased to have read her book thank you so much for your insights. Yes the outer mirrors our inner and this is a good way to learn about yourself. If you are having difficulties in life seek out help it's easier to have assistance; when you decide to heal yourself. Be mindful of your beliefs are they yours or others is it time to reassess your beliefs? Leah can help you to take the right path to your self improvement. Thank you for your insight Leah. Christine C.

Thank you, Leah. To say I have enjoyed your book just would not be true. But, to say it has helped to put to bed a lot of feelings and thoughts that I needed to about my first marriage. Also, in having talks and deep conversations with my husband, I feel (we) have brought back a lot of closeness that I - we had lost along the way in our 26-year marriage. So, I want to say "Thank you" for all your help and the book which I would recommend to anyone who maybe in need of it. Patricia C

Thank you to all the philosophical pioneers from the various schools of thoughts over the centuries. Without these people willing to take the risk of going against the thoughts of the time, we quite possibly would be still lost in the Dark Ages

Contents

A Thought 1

What Is Our Matter, More So, What Is Our Body? 3

Our Physical Being 11

How the Mind Alters Health.. 20

A Positive Mental Attitude?
Let's Get Started 28

How Our Beliefs Create Our Well-Being, or Not 39

Tapping 53

What Is the Driving Force of Change? 57

Self-Actualisation 62

One Step at a Time 87

Summary 93

About the Author... 97

About the Book 99

A Thought

Each second of every day, we are in a position to carve a different path. A good friend used to say to me during the worst of my valley experience, 'Now, is the beginning of the rest of your life!' How true it is when you think about it. Each second, each thought, each thing that you do has the potential to change the course of your life. It all comes down to what you choose to move towards, what thoughts you choose to take on at the time and create the actions that support this thought.

Don't let me take away the other side of this reality, which is... It is challenging to make a change; it can be downright confronting, confusing, and hurtful, let alone maddening and all the other feelings you have ever had from childhood. It pays to weigh up the costs of making the difference or not. What costs am I talking about? The cost of self-respect, self-esteem. What does it cost you when you let yourself down, ignore the voice of self-care? What is the cost of the disappointment, frustration, when repeatedly things are not as you would like them to be?

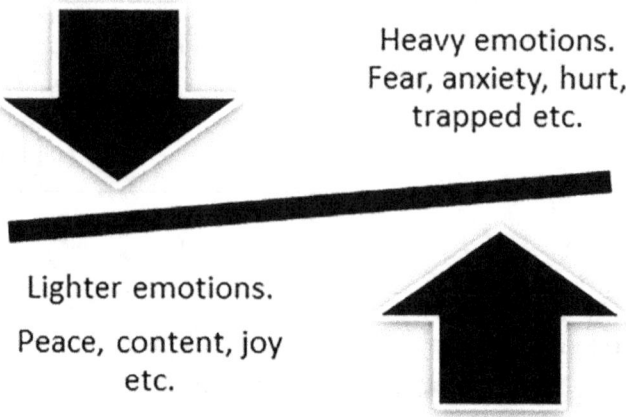

Another cost is the cost of succeeding. Creating the opportunity to make different choices, support and encourage others who choose to change, provide an example of possibility with decision, conviction, and targeted action, create your world the way you want it to be. All decisions are personal, and no one has the right tell another they are wrong or right. We all have free will and choice, and over the coming pages, you will have insight into what tends to make people tick and why we do what we do. The next pages will help you explore what differences you would like to create.

Are you ready? Let's go.

What Is Our Matter, More So, What Is Our Body?

What a question to start with. A few years ago, I read topics on meta and quantum physics, not to the point of getting a degree, but certainly in line with what is matter and what objects, innate or not, are made from. The research clearly shows we are not what we think we are, a solid being that is, as we were taught in school. The topic of size and dimension is considerable, and there have been plenty of good works written to help us lay people understand. Even when reading through the material, it almost seems to be fantasy, but it is there, recorded to our current understanding, and is likely to grow with time and commitment.

The premises of this work are as follows:

- We are not solid, living with solid things, but a set of particles – atoms and sub-particles and a lot of space in between.

- Each particle is vibrating at its own set rate, which determines its position within the periodic table identifying its weight and frequency. Figure 1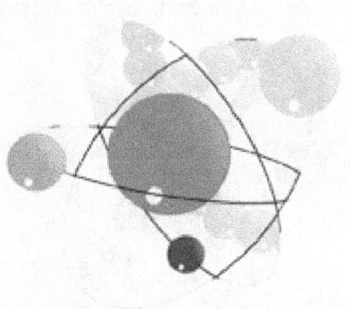

- When particles come together, they create chemical and

structural bonds creating shape, charge, and a vibration signature.

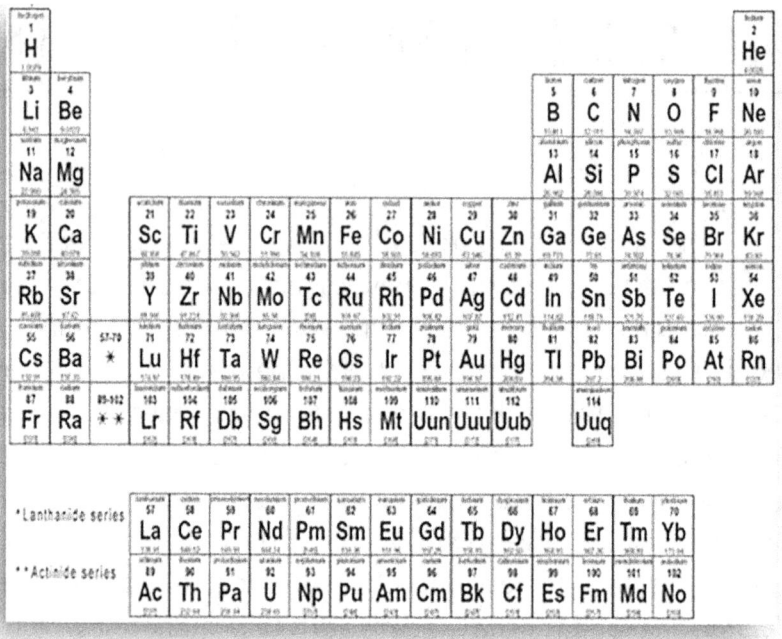

Figure 1 Periodic table

- What we think to be solid matter – our body, the food we eat, furniture, etc. – is the arrangement of these particles in certain a way. Each arrangement has its own vibration. This also applies to our body:

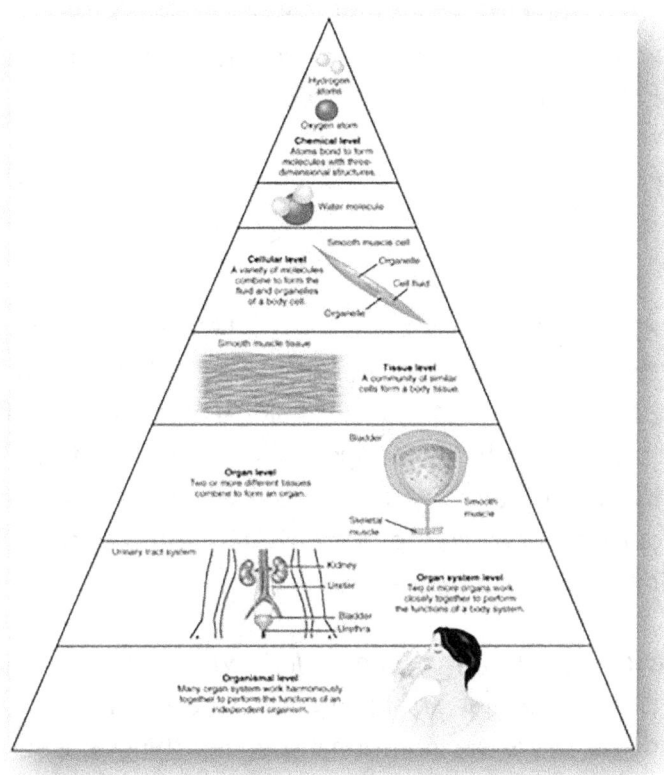

Figure 2 Progressive development of atoms combining to create a human body

The molecular arrangement can also be seen with food. Figure 3 shows the molecular arrangement for glucose, a sugar molecule. The letters represent the minerals. Their arrangement is created by the pull between H – hydrogen, C – carbon, O – oxygen. It's specific mineral arrangement; and it's attraction, repulsion, sharing of electrons with other compounds influences glucose's signature and use. Remember what

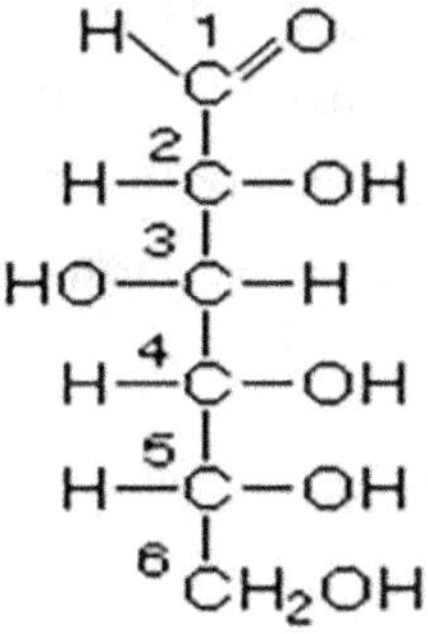

Figure 3 Glucose Molecule

happens when you put various metal objects in a bucket of magnets. They clump together, or they are repelled and join a different clump, or they push some of the objects away.

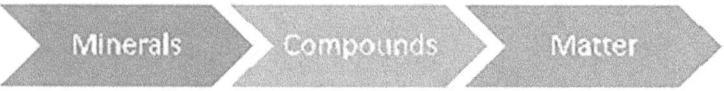

This is the same with nature, minerals interact to form chemicals, compounds and then structures, based on the DNA instructions or blueprint telling the cells how to make things. We see the same principle play out with friendships and relationships, those who we relate with, we are attracted to. Those whom we don't relate to, we limit our time or avoid contact with. This is a very simplistic way of explaining a fairly complex topic.

The individual clumps' or compounds vibration is a set speed based on the molecular arrangement at the moment. One of the influencing factors is the vibrational speed of things it is surrounded by. We see this if we put various metronomes in the same room. While they start at different times, eventually, they swing together at the same speed as the vibration waves create synchronicity. You can see this in action by searching metronome synchronisation on YouTube.

To highlight this even more, we know that each 'thing' has its own signature, as can be seen in Figure 4: the vibration frequency of water, carbon dioxide (CO_2), and carbonate CH_4. They have different molecule arrangements and hence different frequencies.

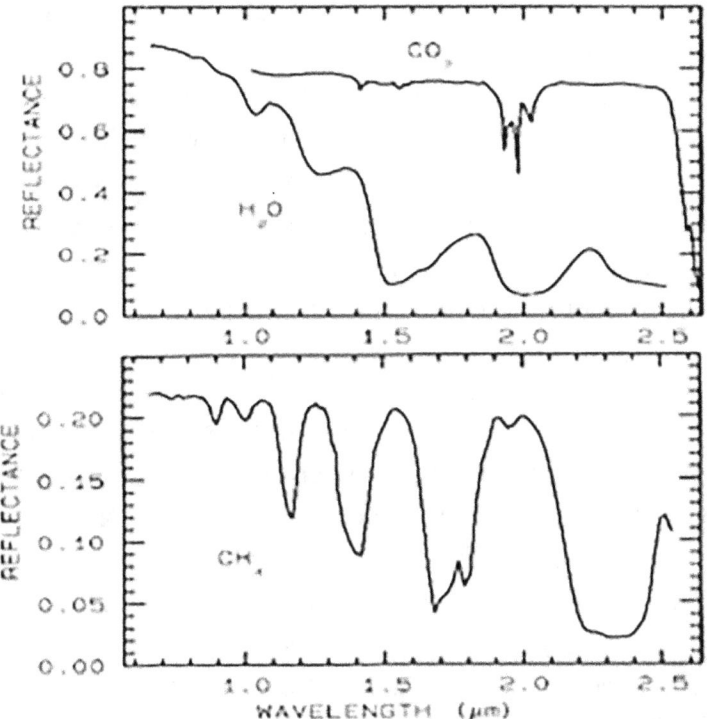

Figure 4 Frequency of water, carbon dioxide, and carbonate

Our body senses what is in our environment, we are constantly reading the temperature, air, food, water – anything that touches our skin. It knows when our body is hurt or damaged any way. This happens when the nerves are activated sending the message through to the control centers of the nervous system or brain. The nerve ends are almost in every part of our body, which is why we can feel and sense so much. Even with the slightest breeze or temperature change, we know it; just as we smell the bakery first thing in the morning, even when it is several blocks away.

Information being interpreted is dependent on a few things – the type of nerve being fired off, as each nerve senses a particular type of information. Each nerve type makes a type of neurotransmitter

- a chemical compound that is released at one end of the nerve and is picked up by the next nerve. When the neurotransmitter activates the next nerve, an electrical charge is generated and moves along the length of the nerve to the other end. The chemical and energetic charge created during this process 'talks' to other cell states in the immediate spaces around the nerve, the body's chemistry, and cross talks to the various body systems. The type of action and reaction is dependent on the nerve cell location and which neurotransmitter is released.

When we 'feel' emotions, it is the emotion's signature chemical structure talking with the cells receptive to the emotion. Our emotions change our cell's function, and body functions. What we 'feel' when we 'feel an emotion' is change in our body chemistry and function at the DNA and cellular level. Emotions are triggered by many things, as you know. Memories, triggers in our everyday interactions, a movie, song, smell, situations, a generational memory held in the DNA. Chemical changes created by food, drinks, and gut microbes, changes in body function, hormones, literally everything change chemical states and therefore emotions change.

> *Everything is an arrangement of mineral ions attracted to each other by their electrons and energy charge. Introduction of other minerals, compounds, chemicals, change its current, pressure, temperature, just as in the chemistry lab experiments the arrangement changes shape and is likely to change function.*

It is the electrons, protons, and their magnetic pull to each other and the frequency the combination then creates. We can see this when we use spectrum monitors which show the various frequencies or energy waves being sent out for each chemical arrangement. It is how MRIs and ultrasound technology help us diagnose changes in the body tissue; it is what we use to blast kidney stones.

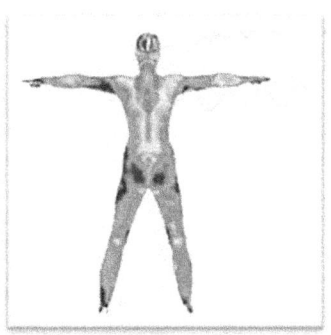

Just as with magnets, the vibration frequency created at any given moment by our body goes out into the environment, and hence, as with magnets, we can attract to ourselves choices that are more in line with what state we are at, at any given moment. The easiest example to highlight this is when you walk into a room and you can 'feel' the type of interaction that was there. An argument that occurred in a room, even after the people have left, can be picked up on. Another example of synchronicity is this: you think about a person or activity, and then out of the blue, that person calls, or you see them or an advertising related to the activity, or you are invited to the activity. The power of the mind/ body to attract people or circumstances to ourselves can be used for good, for lessons, or for even a damn good wake-up call.

We can change our frequency by changing our thoughts, the foods we consume. Different foods contain different minerals and therefore frequencies and our actions – exercise to speed up, meditate, and relax to slow down. It is possible to disentangle the molecular arrangements causing harm by changing our physical, emotional and their chemical state.

In summary, we are made of the same things as plants, cars, water, animals, etc. The defining difference from a structural perspective is the specific minerals used, the minerals' arrangement, and the strength of the attraction. Our body responds to changes in its internal and external environment dependent on the minerals and molecules present at any given moment.

We can create change by making mindful choices of what we put into, onto, and through our body and the thoughts we think, and then act on, letting go of limiting, harmful beliefs that are 'trapped' in our psyche and subconscious body.

Our Physical Being

Cornerstones of Health

There are several layers or influences on our health and well- being. Each is important in their own way, and they interact with each other. Our mental attitude, however, as dictated by our beliefs and values, is the core and primary influencer of our choices, our actions, and therefore our chemistry.

> *Nurture your mind with great thoughts, or you*
> *will never go any higher than you think.*
>
> Benjamin Disraeli

How Your Subconscious Mind Plays Out in Our World

It is quite daunting to start observing our life experiences with a more disconnected eye. To see things, we like and don't like about ourselves and others around us and knowing it all originally began as our body frequency at some time. All things stem from the vibration our emotional self-belief resonates at. Our choices reflection of our self-awareness and perception.

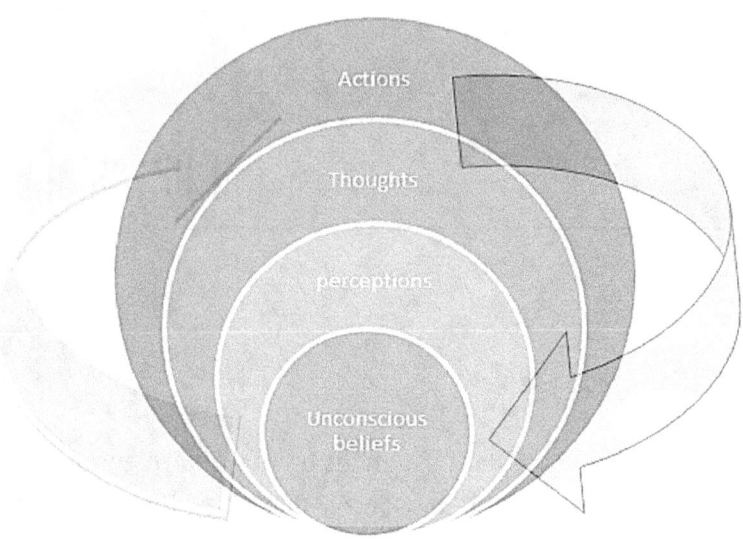

Unconscious impacts on health

Disease Then Is a Culmination of Changes in The Various Layers, a concept that stems from emotional/physical dis-chord through millennium. From early times, people believed dis-ease was an imbalance with spirit and they used various methods to help bring the body and spirit back into balance. It was during the rise of papal Christianity that the church forced perceptions to change around the various pagan beliefs that honored divinity and its sacred wisdom.

When the body is in a state of dis-cord, we tend to be anxious or agitated. Why? There are a number of possible reasons. When we are not in alignment with our highest good we vibrate at a different frequency to our spirit frequency. When we are out of sync, friction is created as our subconscious mind is working towards a set point, and our spirit is working towards another, our body chemistry another. Imagine a three-legged animal and each leg is wanting to go in a different direction. How much fun would that be. It is our duty of self- care to create harmony and being in sync with ourselves. Ideally, we attempt to realign the various parts of our self – mind/emotions, body chemistry, and spirit – into a congruent or united balance.

There are several things that alter our balance. Everything we put into our body with our food and drink; through our skin – body care products, makeup, etc; from the air we breathe; the people we associate with; and what we read, watch, and listen to.

The food/drink we consume is constantly changing our body chemistry at the gut and cell level. All food, when broken down into its nutrients, chemicals, and compounds are absorbed through the intestines, enters the body to be used as building blocks for body function, or body structure, or stored for future use. The amount absorbed is influenced by gut integrity, body requirements, or the immune system's interpretation of what is in the mix.

Harmful compounds can also enter the body and potentially cause havoc.

- If the immune or nervous system is triggered, then the body soon tells you. It can lead to a multitude of conditions from actual diseases such as coeliac disease where the gluten protein triggers the allergic reaction. Seafood and peanuts are other common true allergens. Whenever compounds are seen as a threat, the immune system is fired and the body reacts. This creates disharmony in the body, changing body function, and feelings. The symptoms we feel depends on which part of the immune system is triggered, and the associated changes created. For instance, if histamine is released then histamine symptoms can be created. These include the respiratory, skin, mind, feelings, heart rate, pain etc. This is only one chemical, and a lot of possible symptoms. Imagine what happens if there are multiple triggers firing off at the same time.

- Other reactive compounds can include toxins from bacteria and viruses; chemicals used in farming and food manufacturing; compounds naturally found in foods, such as amines, glutamates, salicylates, phytates, oxalates, and purines; by-products of normal digestive function; and degraded food products from gut microbes. What is in the food, which part of the immune and/or nerve system is triggered, and the way the body interprets the information determine the type of reaction, the symptom, and, in some cases, the actual disease the body creates.

- When the nervous and immune systems are activated, they will over time alter the HPA (hypothalamus-pituitary-adrenal axis). The downstream results are chronic stress, hormonal imbalance, and chronic fatigue. If these occur over a long period, the likelihood of autoimmune (AI) diseases increases. When a person has one AI disease, he/she has a much greater risk of developing other diseases.

Our perceptions/interpretations of events, as well as our primal reactions to the things we see, hear, or experience, trigger emotions and change our chemistry.

- Check in and become mindful of your internal dialogue, conversations with others, emotions that come up for you. Complete the Self-Talk Awareness exercise and gain insight into what you think about things, and drill down till you hear your 'should or rules' about the point in question. From this awareness, you can choose to let go of the unsupportive belief that is potentially causing you harm, modify it so it is supportive to your overall life choices, or keep it, just as it is.

- Another clear indication is the 'in the moment' or 'shouldn't have done/said that' reactions where things are just said or done. If, when you reflect on the situation and it was a 'I shouldn't have' take a step back and consider what you were reacting to and why. Why did you get so agitated and letting go in a way that was bigger than was it bigger your conscious mind could control? Dig deep allow the reasons why rise up and ask for help if it is too big for you to handle by yourself.

- Interactions between our microbes and the food/drinks we consume create acids, alcohols, neurotransmitters, and fermented wastes, to name a few. These chemicals create a change in the intestines and can easily cross into the bloodstream to be transported to the liver, or fire off the nerves and interact with the brain-gut axis and HPA, or even trigger the respiratory system and the heart through the vagus nerve plexus. While the role of gut microbes as a branch of medicine is relatively new, their physiological and biochemical reactions have been known for decades. By targeting microbes, food choices, and how each person responds, we are more than ever in a position to make headway into supporting people with a myriad of conditions, such as skin diseases, respiratory diseases, cardiac disease, hormonal imbalance, liver function/toxicity, autoimmunity, and the like. How? By re-establishing chemical balance and repairing/supporting gut integrity which in turn downplay the immune, nerve, and stress responses triggered by food/drink consumption and microbial function. This relationship is very complex but is providing very positive results for many varied conditions.

Agitation is our body's way of bringing our awareness to what and how our body would rather be or to what our subconscious believes a situation 'should be' or 'could be'. 'The situation' is an opportunity to investigate what, how, and why things are happening and why there is no ease and grace around 'the situation'.

Don't get me wrong. We do need a level of discord to gain clarity along our way to test ideas and to say things are not as they should be. A heightened sense of level of anxiety or 'stress' is not what this is about. The level of discord desired is enough to prompt us to question our lifestyle choices and re-evaluate our 'should and should nots' (though there is no should, but a choice to follow expected behavior or not) and our beliefs and values in relation to what we are reacting to.

Symptoms and diseases provide an opportunity to help us clarify our points of view to ensure we are being our authentic self. It is essential for you to take ownership of this process to help your body and mind reverse the physical formation of unhealthy thoughts, patterns of behaviours, beliefs, or vows. Otherwise, you run the risk of developing more serious diseases.

Well known authors such as Louise Hay, Deepak Chopra, and Dr Wayne Dyer explain this concept beautifully by highlighting the relationships between our subconscious beliefs and the physical/body creating a dis-ease. It is important to comprehend the multifaceted concept of this process. Our thoughts, beliefs, vows, and perceptions of ourselves determine the roles we have in life, how we are to interact in and with, tell the mind to choose. They either create helpful, loving, supporting, and healthy lifestyle behaviours or behaviours that undermine our wellbeing. Hidden, unaddressed, negative experiences can fester and drive our attitudes and choices and develop into diseases if not addressed. This has been seen time and time again in various forms of work.

In summary then, if only one aspect is focused on – the body with exercise and food or the mind – but when we change our food and lifestyle habits or we only take medication and don't address the other supporting factors, such as lifestyle choices, food, and mind, then the problem is only shifted to a different position. The core issues must be addressed to create an ultimate change. These issues are the way we perceive ourselves and our life experiences.

Our Chemical Environment Changes our Chemistry!

Symptoms, however subtle, show up when our body is reacting to the environment in which we live, the toxins and chemicals we are exposed to disrupt our body chemistry, or we are not 'feeling' in oneness with our selves. It is invaluable to question why our body is more sensitive to some compounds than others or why we become agitated or happy or sad or calm in response to different stimuli.

Some sensitivities/reactions can be passed down via our genes which increase our sensitivity to trigger chemicals and situations. Other reasons are our reduced ability to detox and safely remove toxins and chemicals from our body; weaker or more hyperactive immune system, depleted nutrient status and the fact our body just hasn't yet caught up with the chemical swamp our planet is swimming in.

Consider how old the human genome is, a couple of million years, compared to the length of time we have been exposed to a mere 250 years of industrial, chemical, and farming practices compounded by the food and transport industry requiring more and more chemical-laden products. Our body is not up to speed of what these chemicals are, let alone what to do with them.

There is a compounding problem. Many of the chemicals we are now exposed to is killing our natural microbiome, causing significant imbalance and chemical changes within the gastric, respiratory, hormonal, and skin systems. This is leading to increased food intolerances, possibly increased rates of mental health issues, feminisation, and immune system diseases. Disrupted body systems have long-term implications; many without good outcomes.

Microbial disruption isn't the only disruption occurring. Many of the chemicals and heavy metals we are exposed to are disrupting our body functions. They are changing our body chemistry; replacing essential minerals with disruptive heavy metals and altering our biochemical reactions. Examples of this have been known for some time – xenoestrogens are one example where BPA from plastics, mimic the oestrogen hormone and 'tells' the body to behave in a manner that natural oestrogen does. The problem is that oestrogen has a natural rise and fall dependent on our gender, cycle, and what our body needs at a certain time. When we are constantly in the oestrogen 'on' mode, we are at risk of diseases such as breast cancer, visceral fat accumulation leading to insulin resistance, and diabetes. This happens in women. In men, over feminisation occurs with its own complications.

Detoxification

Detox is such a buzzword. We detox our body, our thoughts, our homes; some even detox their email inboxes and detox from technology and some from their friends. There are entire industries dedicated to the process of cleaning out and removing potentially harmful things from our life. What does it mean? In the medical context, detox is

> *the metabolic process by which toxins are changed into less toxic or more readily excreted substances.*

The benefit is obvious. If we don't have potentially dangerous chemicals floating around our body, we are less likely to develop serious conditions such as cancer, inflammatory conditions, and tissue damage. To detox our physical body, we need a variety of nutrients, which are the building blocks of all life; we need to move and ensure the blood is feeding the cells and removing cell waste through the detoxifying organs: liver, kidneys, lungs, and skin. We need to avoid re-introducing toxic foods/chemicals into our body, and it is our duty to do this. Our body is after all ours. We have been entrusted to care and nurture it.

Care is needed when we do a physical detox. The liver has three distinct phases. If we go in too fast and too hard, we can cause more harm than good. We can increase carcinogen compounds if they are not neutralised before they are released into the third phase of the detox process. For more information on how to complete a detox, please contact a functional medicine practitioner or a naturopath so you can be guided safely through the process. It is not a process to play with.

How the Mind Alters Health

Caution needs to be made around emotional associations and environmental triggers. Some have suggested our self-belief and how we see ourselves to fit in the world may 'attract' negative situations or disease symptoms based on our frequency or vibration. We can use this theory to support healing when we ask what the discord is and what lesson we need to consider in the discomfort. What are you holding on to that is not in truth or alignment with what your highest self/love would rather be expressing?

Works in the area of Quantum Physics, the Law of Attraction, and emotional chemistry shed light on the realm as a possibility. It has been shown that what we think, we become. What we believe to be true, is what we experience. Why would it be any different to what our body does? After all, we are constantly awash with our thoughts and self-perceptions. This is a way to explain spontaneous remissions and healings. Are these the results of divine interventions, or is our mind working with our body to explore and heal the emotional aspects of disruption in the body? The imagination, daydreaming & visualisations have power to break through limitations. We have seen this with every new invention, and record-breaking events in history.

Why wouldn't body healing also be about breaking through limiting beliefs? Letting go of the heavy, binding emotions that keep us small? That when we transform them into understanding, forgiveness and love, by letting go of the historic, binding beliefs and heavy energy to be free? This is the premise of the most religious philosophy – to love each other, to have tolerance for each other, to have acceptance for each other, and to love others as we would be loved. This, to me, is the ideology that we need to be gentle, kind, patient, and tolerant to ourselves and help ourselves as we would others to support their life journey.

Holding on to limiting beliefs, ideologies, shoulds, and heavy emotions such as self-flagellation, anger, hurt, and grief does several things. One, it takes a *lot* of energy to keep these feelings in place and hidden so they don't spread through the rest of the body, let alone provide energy to live our life. The energy required to contain these emotions and beliefs sacrifices the energy needed for growth and repair and making lighter emotions such as joy, happiness, and contentment., A metaphysic theory suggests this is how serious diseases such as cancer occur – the dark emotion must be encapsulated so that it doesn't poison the rest of the body, but in doing so, the mutated cells multiply unchecked and have the potential to do serious harm.

> *What you put your attention and focus sets the tone for your whole being in that moment. Be careful then what you focus on, what thoughts you feed, and where you place your energy, as this is what will multiply or increase. What you feed expands. It is impossible to love and hate at the same time*

Our emotions, in essence multiply when we focus on them. Reliving or repeatedly remembering negative situations, feelings, comments, etc., only adds to the heavy, negative body chemistry. Depression leads to a depressed immune system which may not be able to protect the body as well as it could, compared to lighter emotions that produce positive endorphins and support a balanced and healthier immune system.

To focus then on positive things in life expands, and allowing more of the good things to come in. Things such as self-care, enjoyable activities, contributing to things you agree with, and feel good about; doing good for others, practicing gratitude, and being creative, however that works for you all contributes to happiness. These types of actions produce a positive, healthy body chemistry in line with a healthy well-being.

As the saying goes, birds of a feather flock together, which means people are more likely to hang around like-minded people or at least people of similar values, views, and frequency/ vibrancy. Check your friends list. Who do you naturally spend the most amount of time with? What do you talk about or focus on? This gives insight into where your internal frequency is set to. If you like it and it is working for you, then great, keep going. If, however, there is a level of discord, then it is in your best interest to assess, consider, and ask for help to change the internal thoughts into more loving ones, before it is too late. If it means letting go of thoughts, activities, action and people then this is what is needed. It is our duty to be true to ourselves, our calling and to act from our highest good.

Walking away from things and people can be an act of self- love. How, and the intent is the deciding factor in its vibration. All concepts seem very complex, and difficult to sum up into a few paragraphs when there have been thousands of books written describing these thoughts in detail.

> *Our mind is a magnet and we gravitate towards what we think about most. We move towards whatever we have our eyes on.*

There is a saying that goes along the line of 'Forgiveness is for our well-being, not for the other person'. Letting go of negative, heavy, hurtful situations, feelings, and spaces does several things:

- It allows energy to be used for more important tasks such as spending time with people you love and on things you enjoy, detoxing, rebuilding relationships, and finding happiness.

- Overall energy/frequency is raised, lightening mood and increasing contentedness and happiness.

- Life takes on a new meaning as the focus is on things you enjoy and are lighter in nature – love stuff. No, it doesn't mean you will *automatically* attract your life partner, but you may very well attract the people best to help you explore, gain clarity of what you do want, or let go of baggage that isn't serving you so you can move to the next level. Life just seems to be better, and when you come from a pretty dark space, this is an amazing experience and another whole topic in its own right.

- More energy and a lighter body makes detoxification easier when the body isn't so 'blocked up'. Happier people also tend to choose healthier lifestyles of healthier food, movement, and points of view and generally are better rounded.

- A different state of mind and physical environment allows one to be less triggered by their environment. This could be people, emotions, low-quality food, drinks, etc., swapped for more supportive choices which in turn enable the body's chemistry, DNA, and reduce repetitive negative thoughts, which makes more space for self-care, gratitude, and appreciation of the simple things in life.

Is it such a bad thing to self-care and not continually punish ourselves with thoughts, emotions, situations, places, people, etc., that do not co-create a positive and light outlook on life? Yes, your brain and body go with you wherever you are, so physically moving jobs, house, town, etc., may not be the solution but certainly may be part of it. Distancing yourself from negative, hurtful situations, can give you the opportunity to create a very different outlook, connections, and responses. After all, we experience situations by what we bring to it. The other side of the situation is for someone else to be concerned about.

If we are constantly berating, criticising, judging, and doubting ourselves, then it is almost impossible to achieve our goals.

If we are not looking out for ourselves, who will? I ask you then, ae limiting beliefs, self judgement, critism etc a form of self-harm?

Ask yourself this too...." Would I dare talk to others the way I talk to myself?" If the answer is no, then you are self-harming.

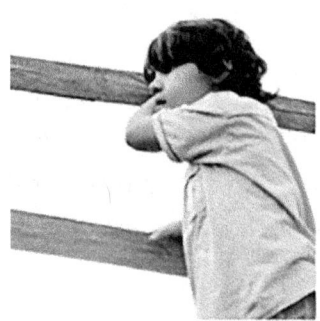

It is essential to recognise how we perceive the world. What is your general perception, negative or positive? A positive mental attitude is essential if we want to live life to the fullest.

What Are We Working Towards?

There is an innate force, an essential ingredient, that drives us towards being the best we can be, towards self-actualisation. We inherently wish to be the best we can be. Children are born innocent, and over time they experience and learn that things are not all innocent and easy. I think we are born self-actualised but go full circle as experiences, learnings, reinforcement, and life happens.

We come to a place in time we need to have a life spring clean out, assessing ourselves to see what we choose to keep, polish or ditch to come back to being the best we can be. Why is one of life's mysteries and depending on which philosophy you work with – Christianity, Spirituality, Buddhism, Taoism, Islam, etc. –the basic premise is that we each ultimately have free will, and the teachings are there to guide us back to the highest, universal power of love. Beyond this, each of us needs to contemplate what the meaning of life has for us.

How do we then come back to self-actualisation? First, we need to live life. The various experiences shared with us by our community, society, family, friends, school, and other adults all leave their mark. Each experience, the good, the bad, the ugly, helps to create and reinforce our reality we choose, our perceptions, beliefs, and expectations.

Considering most of our primary perceptions are created by the age of seven, the early years where we have little direct influence are critical; after this time, we are solidifying our early learning experiences, and then after most are attempting to achieve their life goals and clarify their beliefs and what is important to them.

During adulthood, because we have personal choices, it is our responsibility to become aware of what, how, and why we are thinking, doing, and feeling what we do. We are responsible for parenting ourselves. We are required to take ownership and responsibility as adults to perform, provide, and contribute not only to our lives but also to others'. The biggest gift we can give ourselves and then others is making conscious choices, by choosing from a space of self-respect and honoring our need to experience and heal any previously acquired limiting beliefs.

Accepting or rejecting the various beliefs or patterns we create on a regular basis is to create the type of life we truly would like to live. This is what I would call 'getting real', becoming very clear on what is controlling our feelings, thoughts, and actions and then fine-tuning them to ensure the experiences you truly want to live with.

Sometimes the very first step is to start saying no to the thoughts that come up that are not in alignment with your desired outcome and asking for help to let them go. I am of the view that to make significant changes, it is invaluable to learn techniques of mind change and 'in the meantime' get help. Your thoughts, beliefs, and patterns have been around since your birth if not before, if they have been inherited via your genes so you most likely don't have the skills to make the changes; otherwise, you would have already done so.

We can view life as an opportunity to practice being our highest self, more often than not. Life with all the different characters, personalities, and events playing out simultaneously could be seen as one giant ballpark where each person is a ball flying around through space. We come close to some and are attracted to others like magnets; with others, we may be repelled, again like magnets do, and others we may not have any attraction or contact with. How our 'ball' is what is it made of, how strong the outer shell is, how much magnetic pull does it have, or even how much it pushes the other balls away when they get too close. Balls in this vision are innate without feelings, and so they just fly around bumping into balls and hanging out with others as they come across them. They don't get upset as the various balls move to and away from them. Things are just as they are.

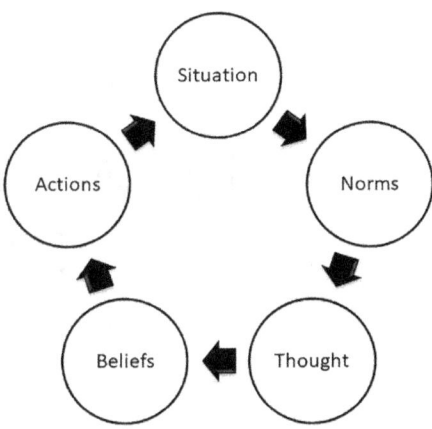

Figure 5 Cycle of Belief and Behaviour Creation

As humans, we have ego and an immature ego tends to have feelings that we associate as 'good and bad'. We see things more in 'black and white' and not so much in grey. Things are either 'this or that' than possibilities. Life gives us a framework to be like the flying balls. We move around, move close to and away from people. We hang out with a few and interact or repel others. It gives a chance to polish up our 'ball' to be what our inner guide wants us to be. The inner guide is love, and when we allow ourselves to operate from that space, we have more compassion, empathy, help, and healthy boundaries. We don't easily allow negativity to come close as we respect the universal laws above ego laws. The outer shell of the ball in this analogy is our ego and personality, our character that we take on or the mask that has been given to us during our childhood.

As we become older, it is healthy to question our ego, our beliefs, and our values. It gives you the opportunity to sift through what is making up your mask, beliefs, and values and choose which parts you wish to accept, keep, and agree to work with or transform any you feel does not represent who you truly choose to be for the belief and character traits you choose to have. In all of this, it is vital to take ownership of decluttering your subconscious mind's filter to make a stand for yourself and who you truly want to be.

A Positive Mental Attitude? Let's Get Started

If you look through bookshops, social media, and self-help messages, you see a waterfall of information dedicated to the mind, perception, and attitude and how these things influence the overall outcome on your life. The latest messages going around include happiness, gratitude, and mindfulness. They can be seen as 'simple' enough to say, but it is harder to work out how to achieve it.

One's self-esteem and self-belief, perception, values, and life views dictate what one's life looks and feels like. These life scripts are messages handed down from one generation to the next – verbal, physical, subtle messages given by people you consider important: parents, other adults, teachers, extended family members, siblings, friends, and workmates, the list goes on. We gather the collective, cultural beliefs, values, etc., which mold the general attitude and behavior of the population.

There are many authors who have written on this topic alone. Tony Robbins, Stephen Covey, Neale Donald Walsch, Brandon Bays, Dr Wayne Dyer, Deepak Chopra, Oprah, Marianne Williamson, Gabriele Bernstein and Brene Browne are some of the good examples of people who have written on how and why life messages become our beliefs and vows we make create an outcome – our life. Better still, these authors go on to explain how to release beliefs and vows that are limiting us. When the limiting beliefs and vows are removed, energy is freed to allow more positive results to follow.

It is important in the context of this book to highlight some premises about this idea. The body is one amazing piece of work and in particular the mind and how we, as individuals, relate to the world around us. The *conscious mind* is the 'brain' part that we are familiar with. The conscious mind has the capacity to process information from the outside world from our senses of taste, smell, touch, and hearing. It is the mind that integrates incoming information, creates concepts, creates ideas, and stores memories of events or information. This is the part most people are aware of because it is just there. We can 'hear' ourselves think, plan, or just critique things happening around us. It is like having a bunch of people constantly with us, talking with us and giving us their view of the world as each sees it. Each voice or person has his/her own role to play in the creation or storage of knowledge, memories, and our overall interpretation of the world we live in. Each has the capacity to think and integrate incoming information from the external environment or from an image or a dream. Information in the conscious mind goes on like a chattering commentary of how things are, and depending on the memory event one looks at, it can have any number of voices giving their opinion about a single event.

These voices arise when our mind decides to give its opinion or interpretation of a situation or a memory. The most common 'voices' are the critic, the analyst, the thinker, and the child. Each is powerful and demands to be heard, and when we ignore them or struggle to acknowledge what they are saying to us, they get louder or, just like a child who is feeling ignored, become more attention seeking and demanding. Over time though, they, like people who are not heard, give up and will not continue to share things with you. This is a dangerous place to get to as emotions, like children, can get up to mischief and cause havoc in your body, your actions, and the magnetic pull you send out to the world.

There are many ways to determine your primary 'voice', and there are equally more titles given to the filters we use. It is the 'voices' that are the filters through which we interpret what we see and hear. They represent our interpretation of the situation, based on our belief system at the time the event occurred. Each one will offer its opinion on the situation at hand, but often one or two of these voices are predominant. This is what gives us our personal characteristics, as we operate from these principles. Complete the Self-Talk, Self- Awareness activity.

The *subconscious mind* is the part of the brain/ body that most are *not* aware of. Often it is sensed via intuition, the gut feeling that may be heard through the voices mentioned above. The subconscious mind is more powerful than the conscious mind as it functions throughout the entire body, in our cells, in our DNA. It is subtler, and many people are not aware of its workings. The subconscious mind holds our memories, beliefs, and values; it can be generational – passed on from one generation to another through the DNA or by living in the beliefs being portrayed by those around us. Life incidents are stored depending on a number of factors.

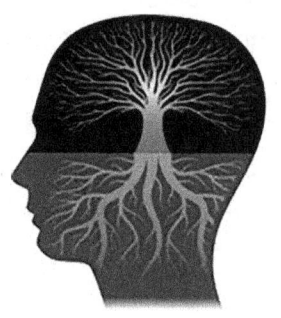

Our five senses take in an amazing amount of information. It is processed in the brain to note what is happening in the world around you. The emotional part is processed at slightly a step behind, however, depending on the intensity of the emotion or the frequency it feels an association between what is seen, heard, smelt, and (touched) felt, and then the memory file is created. All sensory information is matched against previous experiences that have a similar 'theme' and are then stored.

The intensity of the situation from real or perceived danger, intensity of emotions can trigger shutdown or suppression of the memory.

The brain shuts down the memory, sealing it in a closed chamber to protect the person from easy, ongoing recall. Shutting down, or hiding the memory does not hide what happened, or stop the program it creates from running, but stops the mind from remembering the detail of the incident. The body chemical changes are ongoing, and the person may not know why they behave, think, and feel differently; or why they react in ways that is so out of character for them.

The level of emotional intensity the memory recall creates is determined by which 'button' it triggered from the past, similar to which file recall button on a computer program. The click opens up the file, the data is cross-referenced to the data in the current situation, and an automated response can be given.

Memory can be recalled 'as if it was yesterday' when the original incident was charged with emotions and triggered into the conscious mind in two primary ways. When current situations have similar components to the original experience such as sounds, smell, actions, touch, places, seasons etc, or the mind relaxes enough to allow the bubbling memory to pop up out of the blue. The re-playing of the memory is like etching a deeper groove into a record that keeps playing the same song over and over and over again, or the additional, reinforcing data is stored with the file, packing it up a little bit more, reinforcing the theme of the file, such as 'I'm not good enough' and 'These things always happen…' 'I did this or that, and I am therefore responsible for… ' Are these statements true? Are they biased and seen by a limited aspect based on what is contained in the file?

The downside of shutdown is the situation can be buried or suppressed deeply in the person's psyche and body. It becomes a core issue from which perceptions and beliefs are created. Automatic or knee-jerk reactions to similar situations, people, or circumstances, if they are close enough to the original incident emotions associated with the event at the time are triggered. This is the basis of post-traumatic stress disorder, where the core memory of a horrific incident is replayed or triggered by things that have no threat to life but feel or seem similar to the originating incident. For veterans, it can be the backfiring of a car or the chopper flying across the sky. These are just a few examples. Even sleeping and the relaxing of the conscious mind to keep the memories locked in can allow the deep horrific memories to surface.

When there are repeating themes re-enforcing or linking associations made between the events, then a 'file' is created. Each time an event that is similar in nature is experienced, it is unconsciously matched to the file to see how we 'should' feel, interpret, and react to the current event. It can be seen as an onion ring layering or tree rings which with each event or experience that has a similar theme, the person has the opportunity to decide how to interpret and respond.

The subconscious is powerful in influencing our thoughts and actions without our realising what we are doing. It is from the subconscious we innately express ourselves and react to the world and people. It is the place from which we create our personal world experiences. It is that knee-jerk reaction, especially when we have no idea 'why we just did what we did, said, or thought'. These situations are giving us very clear insights into deeply entrenched beliefs.

There are many things that embed beliefs into our psyche, the most obvious being our home environment, school, friends, etc. Anyone or anything that has an influence on or over us has the potential to create a new belief or alter a belief that we currently hold. They are the subtle messages hidden in the words and actions we are constantly exposed to. It can be the hitting, violence, anger, words, actions, or even neglect that sends the message to us. The same is for positive messages, those of love, acceptance, encouragement, support, etc. For most, our primary beliefs are ingrained into our subconscious by the age of seven. Fortunately, though, our beliefs can always be uncreated, changed, reviewed, fine-tuned, or strengthened whether we are aware or not. The longer a belief is held, the stronger it becomes entrenched into the subconscious as experiences reinforce or challenge these beliefs. Just as a tree grows from a seed or a root, our beliefs can grow or be altered depending on the elements the 'belief tree' is exposed to.

We get a glimpse of our beliefs and values in the hidden messages in our experiences. Our self-worth, our self-perception of how and where we fit in the world, other people's expectations of us, and our 'should or should not' rules are encoded in the way we allow to be treated by others, what we react to, and how we react. Engage the action of going third person. Sit in the balcony seat in the theatre of life and explore the scenes, the dynamics, the subtle body language that is going on between the actors. See through the eyes of curiosity and you will gain insight into what is going on, your interpretation that is, and then you can feel into the situation and feel what feelings are coming up for you and just ask 'why'? What is the first time this feeling occurred, do I need to keep this, or what is the lesson that can be taken from this experience?

Thankfully, good feelings also get trapped and are available on recall. Think back to a happy childhood memory. It could be simply swinging on the park swing. Now recall who else was there. Who were you with? Was it a sunny day? How did you feel? What were the feelings you had that day? Can you smell or taste the food you were eating while you were there? What was the message you learnt at the time? Maybe it is one that swinging at the park, with ice cream and family = happiness and love. Each memory depending on its emotional essence powerfully influences our thoughts and actions, often without realising it. Our beliefs, thoughts, etc., can be either positive or negative depending on the messages being given to you by the events around you at the time.

How about this? Do you remember the time you found yourself in the fridge looking for a piece of cake after you had an interesting conflict/ discussion with your partner/friend/child but didn't remember walking over to the fridge? Or the times you got upset and didn't speak your true feelings? And what about the times when you watched TV instead of being honest about the situation and then soon after, you developed a sore throat or a stiff neck or a cold? This is the work of the subconscious mind recreating situations that match feelings or subtle memories of a previous event. Your body is acting out to get your attention because the emotions are playing havoc in your body. What are you ignoring or ignorant to what is there because you are not aware?

Again, it is how we interpret the experience that carries its current influence. It is the work of the subconscious mind influencing your actions. The subconscious is the filter/lens through which all events are viewed. It creates your reality, your truth, but the good news is, it is only a perception and it can be changed. Ask anyone else about what happened in that memory and I bet they would recall it differently.

Life Situations in the Amphitheatre Activity

Each second, we find ourselves in situations which, if you allow your attention to focus on these situations and consider

'What is really going on?'

'What are your thoughts/dialogue around the situation?'

'Who is there with you?'

'What is your interpretation of the situation and consider why the situation is happening to begin with?'

'What is the lesson in the situation, in the dialogue, in the pattern being played out?'

If you are open to looking at yourself, not from a position of judgement but from curiosity, I suggest you do what I call 'going third person'.

It is about allowing a part of you to drift up and watch from a distance, detached and without emotion, as if you were looking at a play on stage. Completing this exercise, you may develop a different perspective of your own reactions and others you are interacting with. You may have a bit more empathy or compassion for the 'actors' in the scene as you can see each actor's point of view with less emotional investment in the situation. This activity gives us the opportunity to consider what and why things happened or are happening and what the other possible choices are in the situation. You can also, with consideration, develop a different perspective and belief around what might have previously been a core belief. You may want to choose a different outcome, and so the 'actors' would need to behave and say different things. As the director of the imagined screenplay, you have the opportunity to role-play various words, themes, and actions and even bring in other actors or ask some to move. It really is very powerful and healing if you allow yourself to venture into other possibilities of thought.

Third-Person Activity

In this exercise, you are the director of the scenario. You are sitting in the balcony of a theatre so you can see all the actors on the stage and hear what is being said. You ask for the memory of the situation in question replay on the stage, in sequence. During this, you will hear, feel, and see what happened, as you recall it. When the scene comes to an end, you get to ask each actor in turn what their point of view and why they did and said what they did. You can talk with them and ask clarifying questions, of what, and why, restating what they said to you. Ask them how they feel and what has been going on for them. You also get the opportunity as if you were really talking to them (calmly), how it was for yourself, what came up for you during the situation, how you felt, and your interpretation of what has been happening and what happened in that instance. The idea is to help them and yourself to understand and see the other person's possible point of view. Ask them what they needed from you and what you needed from them. What needed to be said, done, or followed through with?

After you have spoken with each of the actors, think how you would have preferred the situation to have happened. Who needs to play out the scene or parts of the scene? Does anyone need to leave, or does someone need to come in to the situation? Now, this time move through the situation as you really want it to happen. What did you need to do and say? What did the others need to do and say to help a smooth and lighter demonstration of the situation you are working through?

Notice how different you feel, how they feel. Keep 'developing' the script to create the desired vision in your mind. Just by the power of intent, and voicing your preferred outcomes, and actions, letting go of the attached emotions and expectations of others can create a new set of 'rules' in your subconscious. At the end of each time the situation plays out, ask all present if it is possible to bring them all together to hug and thank them or to have a group hug even. What needs to be said and done from here not to nurture peace and more harmony? When you get to the forgiveness and hug phase individually or as a group, then they are able to leave the situation and the stage. Their work is done on this particular situation.

Completing this exercise doesn't mean you will not get upset, hurt, or annoyed again or that the situation doesn't happen again. What it can mean is each time in the future a similar situation arises, the similar situation can have less power over you. You start to choose different words, actions, and responses because you have started to reprogram your memory bank to what you would like to have happened. This is what successful people do. They see the result, how it will look, feel, smell like, what they will hear, see, and be, as they are moving through the various stages of their growth. Sports people see the competition event first in their mind played out in their favour before they go into the final race. They will perform as they have done in their mind thousands of times beforehand. They have mentally and emotionally started the programming of their mind and body towards their desired outcome.

It isn't always easy sailing, particularly with different elements in real life playing out on life's stage with you; more so because you haven't yet practiced the new steps and lines with them yet. Give yourself patience and grace to have a go, knowing that small changes are being made, because you are choosing to do things differently, and sometimes that is enough to get the ball rolling, so to speak.

When I go to 'third person' and take the time to really 'get' what happened, what I did, said, and felt, and how far back these knee-jerk reactions have stemmed from, I tend to have quite a few aha or lightbulb moments of awareness. Sometimes I feel embarrassed about my behavior, but that quickly shifts to compassion when I see the logic I was operating from in the instant. It doesn't make things 'right'. However, I can see and empathise with myself as to why I would do and say the things I did. I find it even more healing when I contemplate how and why others have said or done some really hurtful things. After all, hurt people lash out as a protection mechanism or a cry for help, or they don't know how to do it any other way. When thinking from these premises, it is easier to forgive and extend a hand of support or compassion than when what I really wanted to do was yell, scream, swear, and hit something, or them.

How Our Beliefs Create Our Well-Being, or Not

Specifically, Figure 6 shows the different components that influence our health, but it is our programming or our beliefs that determine everything else. Figure 7, it is our beliefs, about ourselves that determine the choices we make about self care, food choices, exercise, self-perception; how we look after out thoughts and our mind. These combined influences influence our wellbeing.

Our beliefs, especially about ourselves, determine the choices we make in relation to our self-care, food choices, exercises, self-perception, and how we look after our thoughts and our mind. All these combined influences our well-being. We eat foods that nurture us, we move or exercise, we choose to say no to things that are not healthy for us. We create healthy boundaries that are self-respecting and develop self-empathy, consideration, and support. Our choices for work or our attitude to life in general is positive and uplifting. Positive people who appreciate themselves are achievers, but also gentle when things are not working easily and are gentle on others too as they know everyone is doing the best they can, with the resources and circumstances available to them.

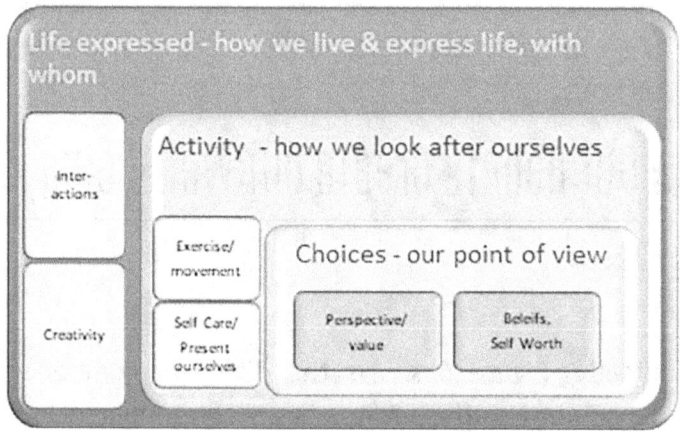

Figure 6 Life Expressed

Decisions serve as the conduit through which emotions guide everyday attempts at avoiding negative feelings (e.g., guilt, fear, regret) and increasing positive feelings (e.g., pride, happiness, love), even when we lack awareness of these processes. (Learner 2014)

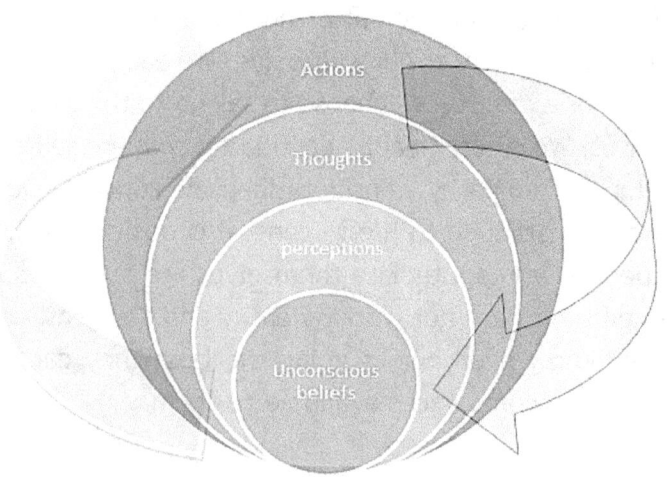

Figure 7 Unconscious impacts on health

If, on the other hand, we have beliefs that 'life is hard' or that 'we aren't good enough', then to fulfil this thought, we make less supportive choices because we have limiting, less-than-best thought patterns. We choose to subtly (or not) self-harm using food, alcohol, drugs, 'bad relationships', exercise, and how we think and talk about ourselves. People tend to blame others for their misfortunes and experiences and live with the victim mentality, asking to be rescued as they are not able to rescue themselves (because they are not worth it).

Not sure where you are at? That is OK. There are a few things you can do to see where and how you see yourself. The first is completing the wheel-of-life activity. This is a global view of where and how you see your life.

Wheel of Life Activity

It helps to start at the global level, to take time out and review how you see/feel your life as you are currently living it and see how the various parts of your life are playing out. It is an invaluable tool to assess how you feel your life is in different areas such as relationships, health and well-being, work, and achievement, among others. Read through the material on the wheel of life and complete the assessment. The answers can help uncover where, how, and why you might choose to make positive changes into your life.

To start determining how you see yourself, it might be as simple as asking yourself two questions. Listen to the very first thought that comes to mind. These thoughts are the most honest. Do not evaluate the responses or judge them. There is no right or wrong answer; it just is.

- Where on the scale in this segment of my life do I fit?

- What level would I like this segment of my life to be?

Use two different-coloured pens or different marks to know in a few months' time your original assessment. By considering where you feel you are at now gives you something concrete to work with. Remember, awareness is the first step, and with a limited or unconsidered response, we let ourselves down. It is like wishing on a star, without knowing which star the wishing star is. Other questions to ask are

- How do I feel about myself?

- Why do I create negative experiences if I don't like them?

- Why do the same things seem to keep happening to me?

- Why do I start eating better and then only within a time 'go off the rails' and resume unhealthy habits again?

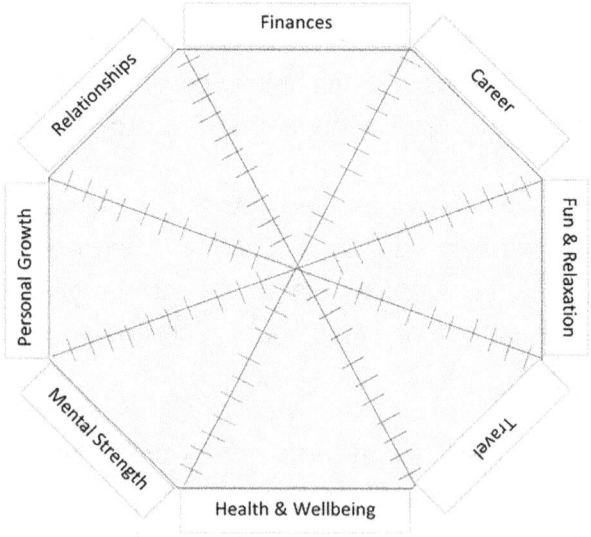

Opposite Hand Writing Activity

A helpful technique is *Opposite Hand Writing* - to write the question in your prominent hand, the hand you normally write with, and use the other hand write the answer. You may not be able to read it easily, but it helps the brain release the real belief behind the question. For more details, see Michael Rowland's *Absolute Happiness: The Whole Untold Story* (1994). The other is to complete the 'third person' activity outlined earlier.

Ask for help from a counsellor, hypnotherapist, or kinesiologist and choose a style of therapy you feel comfortable with. Work with them to help uncover your current truths as you see them, and then transform them into beliefs that you would rather have.

The questions of 'why' and 'how' a situation/food choice/habit makes you feel are very powerful. If you can, sit and continue to ask why and how questions until you get an emotional response, then ask a few more times in that vein and you *will* find the underlying answers. For instance, I feel at times frustrated by my lack of interest in some activities. I then will work through the layers of the feeling and get to what is it that is driving the emotion of frustration. Let me show you:

I am feeling frustration around this project. What is at the core of this?

- How can I be worthy or be able to make a difference when I am so small compared to the 'big names' in the industry?

- Who would listen to me? I have no formal qualification, only life experience, tons of therapy and lots of reading, courses, etc.

- Who would trust me to make a difference in their life?

Thank you for sharing these things. What else is going on?

- Others seem more committed. I don't feel committed to the big picture.

- I'm scared of getting it wrong.

- I'm scared of hurting someone, of being pointed at.

- Can I really make a difference?

What else is there? What is under these thoughts?

- Who am I to be in this position? I am just me.

What else is under this?

- It is safer to stay small. I am less likely to be victimised or singled out.

- I can't get it wrong if I am not doing anything.

- I keep changing direction, and this seems to be fraud, instability, and stupidity. (Wow, this is a new one.)

What else is under this?

- I just want to get by and be OK. Safe, not stand out, and small is OK for me.

(Now I know I am getting to the truth of what is keeping me where I am. There is a level of vulnerability and caution felt in my body. It feels like 'OK, this is how I see it.') A frank and honest conversation is being had. I also feel embarrassed that I have accepted this for so long, but also while I look back over my current life to date, I see the pattern, the times I have repeated behaviours that have kept me safe – studying instead of working, saying no to offers that would have brought me out and allowed me to use my skills, and sabotaging opportunities and lessons because of the things deep inside me.

I know my background, and I have been victimised many times over for standing out, attempting to make a difference, and supporting the underdog. I am aware that the word 'safe' is used often in my vocabulary, and this is a big part of my life. While I can't really recall any significant event in this life, past life therapy has shown many a time when I have been killed and needed to go into hiding to protect myself and my family. This realisation is the root of my frustration with myself. I am frustrated that I would rather stay small and hidden – I actually live in a cabin near the beach and have very few neighbors around me. It is in a secure park so people can't just 'rock' up. I can see how this deep-seated belief is playing out, and to move forward, I know it needs to be transformed into a positive state. I like to ask for help on deep historical issues when they come up. It is much easier and more permanent. Personally, I have a select number of therapists who work with me and my 'history'. (They have always turned up in my life at the right time and in the right way.)

How Our Self-Perception Controls Our Life

If we don't love ourselves, we are less likely to care for our body as much as we do other people or things. We tend to make less-than-loving choices, put others before our own needs, sacrifice and be a martyr, or be overly self-critical, self-abusive, self-neglecting, etc. We tend to make choices that have instant gratification over useful choices to help us feel good about ourselves and not invest in the longer-term outcome. Quick fix is a motto in its own right.

Ask yourself, 'how often do I ask for what you actually need to support me? There is a difference between desiring chocolate, alcohol, caffeine, etc., because it tastes good and doing harm by indulging in excess. Do we support our body function with adequate rest, relaxation, nutritious foods, exercise, stress management, etc., or do we push ourselves too hard, too long, and feed it foods and drinks that can cause harm? If we crave something, it is like a red flag for us to look at something from a different perspective. There seems to be a real link between what we crave and a deeper message to be looked at. That is what I have observed with clients.

When we

- choose to ignore our body and the subtle messages and push on no matter what, we are in effect self-abandoning;

- push our emotions aside or ignore the warning signs, we are self-neglecting;

- consciously choose to eat poorly, drink too much, take drugs, etc., we are self-harming; and

- talk badly about ourselves and verbally/mentally criticise and bully ourselves, we are self-abusing.

If we were to treat others the way many treat ourselves, would we be charged with assault and abuse? So, if we wouldn't do these things to others, why would we do it to ourselves?

There is a saying, 'Do unto others, as you would have done to you.' The point of this statement is to look at how you are treating yourself because this is how you expect to be treated, and more than likely, it is how people are treating you. The world is a like a mirror, and as much as it can be difficult to see what is being thrown back at us, often, what we whine about or comment on reflects what we are doing to ourselves. Harsh words, but I encourage you to think about it.

By giving in to others, bending over backwards, etc., we show how we would like to be treated, but do we look after ourselves in the same way? Would we encourage a tired parent to keep working hard or suggest they take some time out to sit and have a cuppa or even play with the children to invest back into the family? Do you say to them, 'The house is a mess, so you had better get off your tired backside and get on with cleaning up to shine (only to be messed up again tomorrow so you get to do it all again)'? No, I will bet you would suggest, 'The house isn't that important if everyone is healthy and that another day isn't going to hurt. You will feel better and get it done faster anyway after a good night's sleep.' I'm not saying not to do things ever. I am suggesting to honour how you feel, get help in the ways possible, and schedule and engage others to help if possible. Not always easy, I know, but it does make a difference.

Take note of what you are telling yourself. When your 'should do this' voice comes up, be sure to ask why, and really think through what you would tell your best friend when he/she are in the same predicament. If it is a softer suggestion and is viable – honestly, then take the softer version. Thank the voice that flips the view so you can start to look after yourself and not harm yourself, again.

Emotions and beliefs, in particular the heavier ones reflecting self-belief and self-perception, and reactionary emotions such as anger, frustration, rage, etc., require a lot of energy and therefore nutrients to keep them contained/safe in the body and not let out. The body will protect itself from potentially harmful, hurtful, or difficult situations. In doing so, the body can trap the negative emotions and our true feelings at the cellular level, altering DNA function, body chemistry, and function, let alone how we see the world. It is worth giving the mind permission to feel and acknowledge the feelings as they come up and learn how to heal them in a safe way. Quality therapy and meditation therapy to express your true feelings around situations, forgiveness exercise, reframing, etc., can all go towards helping you transform your emotions. If at any stage though your emotions are overwhelming, do get help. Lifeline in Australia or something similar elsewhere to talk things through is vital. You don't need to be alone in the journey.

This is why it is invaluable to recognise the emotions in the instant they are there and let them out, in an appropriate manner. I am not advocating hitting or throwing things around in anger or rage but acknowledging this is how you feel, walking away, and dealing with the emotions at hand, then coming back to re-engage when you are clear and talking from truth and not reaction – to make, feel, and express them. Each emotion has a right to be present. It is what we do with them that makes the difference. Big stuff usually means big emotions that need a safe place for them to be.

Talking Gently Exercise

Think about the various parts of your life and consider the things you say to yourself that you should do or the connotation you give to yourself. Then, in the next column, say what you would to your best friend, whom you love and for whom you only want the best.

Your frequent self-criticism statements	What you would say to your best friend

Common scenarios for prompts, if you need them:

- Helping the children with their homework
- Cleaning the house, the car, or your own bedroom
- Using the latest trend in foods, cooking, utensils, etc.
- The way you dress
- The type of work you do
- Financial issues
- Having it all together (or not)
- Interactions with various family members' activities or social events
- Level of activity, fitness, wellness, etc.
- The size of your TV or the number or types of gadgets in the house
- Being minimalist or organised or functional
- Having/not having it all together
- The type or number of things you do in a day
- Having to say yes or no to people
- Signing up for everything even though you don't want to or have the energy to

- Hanging out with the right people, the right social group, the right connections, etc.

- Not speaking your truth in case, you hurt their feelings, even though you are gutted or feeling hurt yourself

- Putting others before your needs, wants, or desires

- Filling up everyone else's cup and being left with the dregs or, worse, dry dust

OK, take a big breath. For many, this is big stuff and can certainly keep us trapped and playing small. We have been taught at an early age to be critical, and I am sure our parents and other adults meant every word with the intent to help us improve, be organised, and have the skills to survive in the world as they saw it. After all, we all talk from our point of reference, and we all mean well when we give suggestions to others, helpful or not. Our intention I am sure is to help and not harm. The unfortunate part is we can cause more harm than not and more so when said in a stressful manner or when the child is feeling vulnerable.

Keep breathing. Now is the time to forgive. Forgive yourself for perpetuating the hurt, without realising what you were doing. Your critic, which learnt very early what and how to say things, has only been doing its job.

What are the top 3 situations that are really not helping you achieve your current change goals?

_____

_____

_____

What is the hidden message in what you hear yourself telling yourself to do?

_____

_____

_____

What other re-enforcing situations or patterns make you believe this statement must be true?

_____

_____

_____

Are you ready to shift it?

Are you ready to talk with yourself as you talk with your best friend with compassion and understanding of how difficult it is to get all this stuff done in your life and how alone you feel at times?

In most cases, you have taken on other people's beliefs and expectations of how things should be done, look, be said, be acted out, or even feel. That is a lot of baggage that you are carrying around that is most likely yours. Is now the time to give some back to the people who gave (forced) these beliefs to you?

Is now the time for you to look at each one individually and choose which ones you want to keep, modify to suit you, or just throw out? If that is a yes, then let's get on with it and start to notice how much lighter and easier things can be.

There are two easy ways to move through, and for the big stuff, like what you are doing here, it is to do both. That is, tap it out and the forgiveness mantra. You are forgiving yourself for taking on hurtful beliefs, but you were too young to know what you were doing when you accepted what was being told to you, and you trusted and loved those who were telling you these things, or you were terrified that if you didn't do what they taught you, it would cause harm. Whichever way you picked the ideas up, know that you were likely not fully aware or developed, and so you are off the hook. Ready?

Tapping

Tapping uses acupuncture points Figure 8 to help release the anchored emotions to the memory, belief or thoughts that come up in the moment. By acknowledging the feeling and/or situation that comes up and finishing the statement that you unconditionally love yourself, or forgive yourself, or honour yourself, or even all three, that you unconditionally love, forgive, and honour yourself, no matter what.

Allow the associated feelings, thoughts, memories, sayings, or voices to come up as you tap your way around the points. There may not be many at first, or there could be a lot. Either way, it really doesn't matter, and there isn't any wrong way to do this. The power of intent is magical, and often starting the process of working towards self-care opens up the opportunities and lowering of the anxieties around it. The second is the forgiveness mantra.

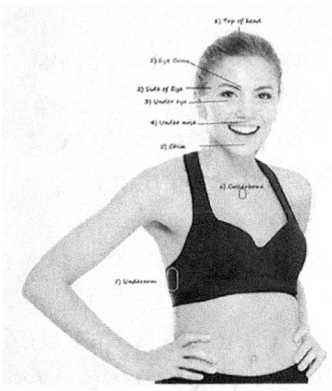

Figure 8 EFT Tapping Points

> *Holding on to resentment is like drinking*
> *poison and expecting the other to die.*

Again, this process is about forgiving yourself for your part in actions or thoughts playing out. You have only been doing what you have been programmed to do, and you have been doing a fine job at that. However, you now have the opportunity to change the belief or the actions to help you live in a way that is authentic to you and what you choose for you.

The mantra is

I forgive you I'm sorry
Please forgive me I love you

is suggested to really move into the experience by visualising the person/s or situations that come up in memory and feel the feelings that were there at the time. Repeat it until you feel full and lighter and hold your self-image in your mind's eye and repeat it again as many times as you feel it needs to be said directly to yourself.

Some of the things that can occur doing these exercises are as follows:

- Feel of being happier, lighter

- More calmness and peace about past events

- Improved communication or acceptance with those who came up in the event's memory

- Better sleep, easier to choose self-care

- Easier to complete the tasks that are important and be OK to postpone the activities that don't serve you

Allow the feelings to come up and acknowledge them without judgement. They will leave easily the more you see them, thank them, and forgive the situation they were attached to.

The magic of the mantra comes from the energy and intent of the words spoken:

I forgive you – transforms resentment and similar emotions you have towards the person

I'm sorry – ignites compassion for the story generated to keep the belief and associated actions in place

Please forgive me – requests compassion and forgiveness from others or yourself for the situations and the harm experienced over time

I love you – is the healing balm to all involved. How relieving it is to truly feel love and connection with others when you have honestly resolved a conflict or supported them through a difficult situation. To say I love you to someone, including yourself, is the most healing feeling, pouring peace and connection through your entire body. Who doesn't love that feeling?

Detox and Our Emotions

Emotions alter cell function by their chemical nature. By undergoing a detox, we change the chemical environment in the cells, tissue, and organs and encourage the release of waste products. This also alters the chemical environment and affinity for the heavy emotions to stay attached to the DNA, cells, mitochondria, etc. A detox enables emotions to come 'free' from the DNA, and one reason why people feel different when they eat well is that their body is undergoing both physical and emotional releases. The simple act of cleaning out the body enables the mind and body to also let go of 'stuff'. This side effect often isn't spoken of but addressed by encouraging people to incorporate meditation, exercise, or other stress management techniques into the treatment protocol. What you do or engage in will be influenced by your personality and what you feel comfortable doing. Whichever method you use to support your emotional healing, it is better to start than not.

In the metaphysical world of mind/body relationships, each organ has its own energy/emotional vibration and hence holds the emotion that matches them: liver – anger and bilious feelings, pancreas – joy, legs – moving forward, and so on. So, when parts of the body are out of balance, we can go in with a general awareness and ask questions more directed to the situations or patterns showing up in your reality.

What Is the Driving Force of Change?

This is a deep question and one that may not be explained in detail in this script. If one reads the great masters of change, the consensus there is an innate 'calling or driving force' that discerns between right and wrong and what our own divine path is. We have already touched on belief systems, the law of attraction, and how we create our disease as a means to become aware. This section is expanding on these topics.

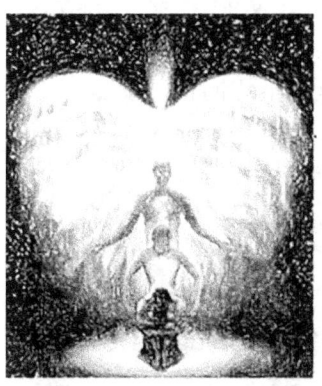

In essence, in our heart of hearts, we know what we have been called to do, because it is engraved into the very core of our being. From an esoteric/ spiritual point of view, it is as in the picture where there is a universal 'knowing' of information that is purity and love. It flows through all of us, and as we have free choice and a conscious mind, to make decisions on any topic about who we are in relation to the situations at the time.

Polarity is in everything: light/dark, love/hate white/black, heavy/light, etc. We have the ability and the right to choose which side of the continuum we live our lives, and this isn't always easy, and is a personal interpretation on spirit.

This aspect of theory also moves through Eastern and Christian philosophy, it is easy to see similarities between them. The bottom line or the most distinct common thread is that love is the highest vibration, from which connects everything and everyone. It is a state of ecstasy, which can be attained in our earthly life. It is really possible to have heaven on earth, well, at least a glimpse or sense of it: tantric sex, kundalini, meditation, prayer, new-born babies, puppies, nature. When we let our 'guard' down, we can see the wonder and the vibrancy of the purity. These are a few instances when we can go into a state of ecstasy and bliss that is mind blowing and so expansive we are everything and there are no physical boundaries.

It is when the body and mind are out of synch with divinity, when our body is not living its divine intention and is not operating from the space of love, or wonder, that there is discord (emotional unrest) or disease (body not at rest). Both have varying levels of being out of balance, and usually it is the emotional discord that begins the change and the mind shuts it out or down for any number of reasons. The longer we 'fight' the feeling and ignore, avoid, deny, dismiss, shut down, or fight against, it can grow. Just like a piece of sand in an oyster creates a pearl, the constant emotional irritation lingers, and the body needs to protect the irritated area until it can no longer go unnoticed by the physical body.

In line with the theory of self-actualisation, divinity only wishes the best for us, to create from a space of love, to live a life that is fulfilling, love filled, and content. Over time though, we create layers of self- *beliefs* then these over times these beliefs have a magnetism of their own. What we live through and perceive is from the layers of self-beliefs and perceptions. These are what we are projecting out there and attracting back to us to experience, see, and feel who we think we are, not what we are.

The more layers there are on the same theme, that we are not love and light, the heavier the experiences, increasing the likelihood of depression, anger, rage, frustration, etc. Our spirit self still perceives others' spirit, but ultimately, we are drawn to people, situations, and reactions based on the beliefs that we acquire with time.

Your subconscious works on creating within your physical world *your* perception of your truth. Your health, your relationships, or your job status changes to reflect *your* true self-perception. The world acts as a mirror to your innermost beliefs. This is most potently seen in relationships. How does this happen? Based on the law of attraction, what we resonate or vibrate at energetically goes out into the world, just as a radio station sends out information for the receiving antennae to pick up.

When we look at various parts of our life, I suggest to look back to your wheel of life and walk around it again and contemplate the 'good' and 'not so good' parts of the wheel. There isn't judgement or emotion attached to this emotional exercise, go third person, and see what is going on. Consider how you feel or the thoughts that have come up while reading this book and doing the exercises. Contemplate if there are patterns, if situations are there that are asking you to look at what you reconsider the way you feel about yourself, or if you reframe and see the other person's point of view or go third person, or even rewrite the stage script on various situations, various aha thoughts that come to mind. You may feel very justified in the way you feel or behave, but is it helping you, is it making your life easier, harder, more or less painful, exciting, light, and a

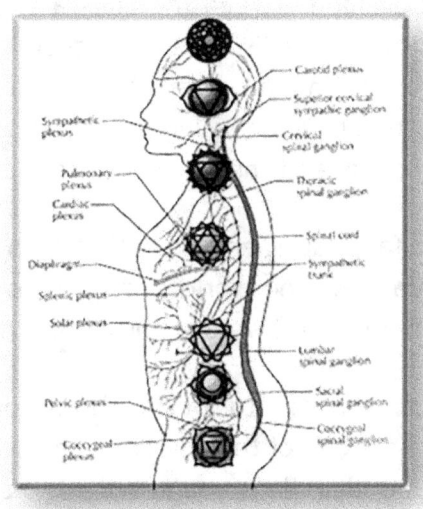

Figure 9 Relationships between the charkas and the autonomic nervous system

positive adventure? Consider your part in what is creating the situation, your point of view, the various times in history you have had similar things happen.

These activities are helpful if you can be honest with yourself. If the feelings are just too big to deal with, or if you are not sure what it all means, get help. It is much better for the layers to be released and healed so that you come back to you and heal well.

Keep in mind too, it can take years of conscious effort of being honest and peeling away the parts of us that have accumulated over our years of life to date.

When we consider the similarities between the theory of self-actualisation or psychology and Christianity, religion, and Eastern philosophies of Buddhism, Taoism, and Hinduism, they all propose the idea that one is innately programmed to improve or progress to a 'higher' level or become a better adjusted individual. Caroline Myss, in her book *Anatomy of the Spirit*, clearly describes the relationship between the chakra system, religious beliefs, and the physical – body diseases that occur when the mind and body are not operating from a center of love and truth. Figure 9. This is further examined by Anodea Judith in the book Eastern Body, Western Mind: Psychology and the Chakra System as a Path to the Self.

It is a fascinating area, one that both unites the various philosophies from around the world and gives us real-life indication of possible outcomes when we are not true to ourselves.

We can continue to overlay the various 'parts' of the body with the nerve clusters of the autonomic nervous system, acupuncture points, and meridian lines and see the crossing over of the philosophies in the physical body. If you take it one step further, consider the disease clusters, cell line divisions, and embryonic division development, and it becomes easier to conceive the intimate relationship between divinity, chi or qu, emotional blockages, and the creation of disease. Table 1

Maslow's Steps	Functions	Chakra Centre	Emotions
Basic survival Breathing, food, drink, sleep, sex, excretion	The living body and its healthy function	Root Base of spine, coccygeal plexus	Fear; Goal: Stability, grounding, physical health, prosperity, trust To be here, to have
		Sacral Abdomen, genitals, lower back, hips	Fluidity, pleasure, healthy sexuality, feeling, function, To feel, to want
Safety and security Economic, social, vocational, psychological	Getting on in the world	Solar plexus Vitality, spontaneity, strength of will, purpose, self-esteem	To act
Belonging and love Family, friendships, intimate connections	Connected to the outside world and others, 'Where do I fit'	Heart Balance, compassion, self-acceptance, good relationships	To love and be loved
Esteem Self-esteem, confidence achievement, respect for others, and respect by others	Being OK with self and sharing ideas, talents, etc., with others in a beneficial and considered manner	Throat Communication, creativity, and resonance	To speak and be heard
Self- actualised – enjoy life in general and in all aspects	Centre of head, at brow level; pineal and pituitary glands; 'third eye'	Intuition, imagination, vision	To see
	Top of head, cerebral cortex	Awareness, Wisdom, knowledge, consciousness, spiritual connectedness	To know

Table 1 Comparison between Maslow and Eastern philosophy based on the chakra system shows the different steps in the ladder towards self-actualisation or spiritual beings

Self-Actualisation

There is a large body of evidence showing habitual thoughts and emotions determine our level of health and quality of our life. While depression, disbelief in one's self, and negative self-talk have a negative impact on health, the opposite is equally true. A positive mental attitude stems from an innate drive in all living things to be the best that they can be - self-actualisation. This journey is a unique personal experience based on our interpretation of our life events and experiences.

Ultimately, self-actualisation begins by taking personal responsibility for your own mental and emotional state, your life, your current situation, and your health. It is the notion that we are entirely responsible for creating our circumstances, health, financial position, relationships, etc., from our own imaginations, beliefs, and thoughts. When we are in alignment with what is the highest and best for us, then life is so much easier. It is like living in another world of possibility. There is a lot less stress, less reactivity, and more responses to life. We get to create what we desire, if it is in our interest. It is really amazing!

Life is full of events that are beyond our control; however, we do have control over our response to these events. Our attitude and self-perception have a big impact on the way we view and respond to all of life's challenges. You will be much happier, healthier, and more successful if you become clear of what your filters (perceptions) are and release the hold of non-supporting beliefs have over your life. Clearing unhealthy beliefs and vows naturally creates a positive mental attitude. From this we can move more easily towards becoming self-actualised.

Self-actualisation, the desire to be the best we can be, is a concept developed by Dr Abraham Maslow, the founder of humanistic psychology. His theories of self-actualisation stemmed from his research of healthy people over a period of more than thirty years. His theories are well supported, and many researchers who have investigated the common threads of very successful people support the basic principles of self-actualisation. Maslow researched the traits of healthy, successful individuals and found they are motivated towards self-actualisation. Ongoing actualisation is

- the reaching of potentials, capacities, and talents as fulfilment of a mission/call/fate/destiny or vocation;

- a fuller knowledge of and acceptance of the person's own intrinsic nature; and

- an increasing trend towards unity, integration, or synergy within the person.

In other words, healthy people are driven to be all that they can be! Maslow is a foundation leader from which many branches of positive psychology, mindfulness, meditations, and health coaching have stemmed from with the premise of helping others to develop their innate resources and talents.

From a psychological view

Over the course of time, many theorists have proposed similar progression from the ego, or simple thoughts, to one that is more secure and caring for the greater good.

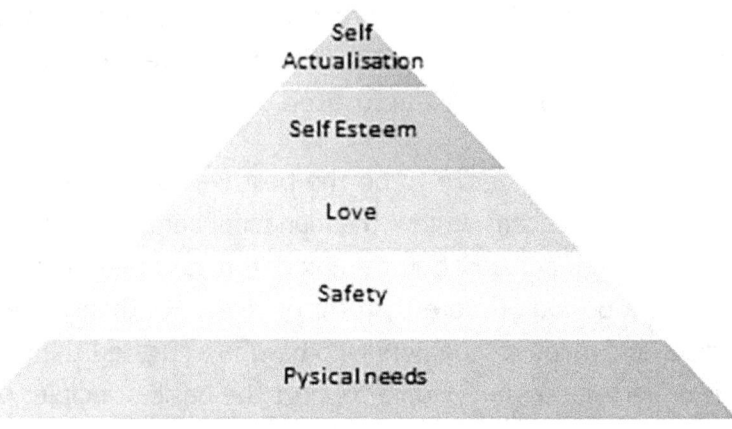

Figure 10 Maslow Hierarchy of Needs

Maslow is known as the originator of self-actualisation, yet there are several crossover theories through the various religious/spiritual schools of thought that also support the notion of moving from a base level to higher levels of awareness. Figure 10

Another basic premise of Maslow's theory is the sense of security as the base or foundation of one's life is essential before being able to move to the next level. The movement through the layers is dynamic, and not a linear line Figure 11. All the best-made plans are still responsive to real life commitments, emotions, other people's needs and expectations, emergencies, personal growth to move into the chosen reality, etc. Life at

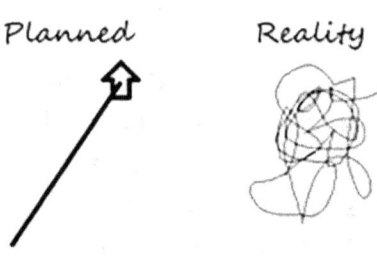

times seems to get in the way; however, it is only doing what it does best – giving us the opportunity to get clear of what we want and what is important to us and we get to fine-tune our beliefs or get rid of the ones that don't work for us anymore. This is actualisation working in us and for us at every given moment, creating the space for clarity and truth, living our lives to the fullest as we desire and choose it to be.

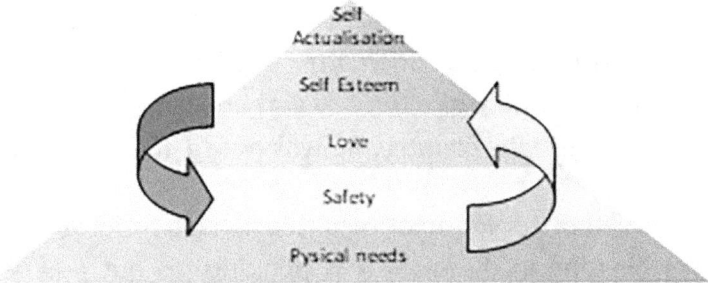

Figure 11 Growth is circular, moving between layers.

Self-Actualisation is not a linear progress up the mountain, and we can be working on the various levels at any given movement depending on what is happening in our mind and response to life as it is happening. For instance, if we feel safe or have a safe haven of home, and for friends to come back to, we are more inclined to increase our adventures and risks – knowing we can come back to our safe zone, if and when needed. As we prove to ourselves and grow along the way by letting go of previous limiting ideas – increasing our confidence, increasing our skills, or gaining recognition from self or others – we continue to progress up the mountain. During times when things are being challenged, when things or people are not doing 'what they are meant to do', it can be a blessing in disguise. The situation is giving us the opportunity to be clear in our intent, our thoughts, or our self-belief and let go of limiting thoughts, beliefs, and people if need be to keep moving ahead. It can also be the universe is protecting us from unseen harm in the future, as described in this folk tale.

> *There was a farmer and a son. Now the son was sickly as a child and didn't grow so strong. Nonetheless, he helped his father with the farm and made up for*

> *his ill health by being a great horseman. One day he fell off and broke his arm and limited his ability to work the field. Now, the father needed to tend to the field, and the son felt embarrassed about being kicked off his horse. Soon after this incident, the war broke out, and while the boy was eager to go and do his part for the country, he was not fit to go to war.*

The moral of the story? Sometimes things happen for a reason and can be a blessing in disguise. It is our duty to put our best foot forward, make our plans, and act on them as we can, then let it go. What will be will be, or *que sera sera*. Not necessarily easy if we feel we need to be in control of our choices and circumstances. The more we attempt to maneuver the various parts of our life, especially the parts that are out of our circle of influence, we tend to push our stress response. Let go and let God work it out on our behalf as it actually needs to be. Heal your emotional responses to the various things that do or don't happen; learn the lesson so that you don't need to do it all again with another situation.

This is not always simple, and as we circle through the loop, the spiral can go up down or keep spinning like a spinning top as we attempt to get our head and heart around the changes needed to ultimately achieve what we want. Sometimes some really hard, honest questions, answers, and actions are needed. However, this is beyond the scope of this book.

Like any skill, the more we practice and get more skilled at the process/action, the easier it becomes. It is possible to be working on several layers at one time and be OK with it. Interesting too is that we become more adept to this, even the 'big things' in life such as the rug being pulled from under us and unexpected left field experiences. While they certainly can throw us, it has been shown more actualised people show greater resilience to life's tests and rebound sooner and stronger because of them. There is a saying 'What doesn't kill us makes us stronger.' Another saying, which I prefer, is 'We are only given what we can handle'. So, the bigger the deal, the closer we are getting to being more complete, and that is exciting.

Mindfulness

The now trending activity of mindfulness, the Happiness Movement, and living in the now also share the same principles. This branch of psychology encourages people to become present in the moment, relaxing the mind to a neutral state, allowing breathing to move more feelings through the body, and facilitating peace and relaxation within the body and mind.

Mindfulness teaches the principle of meditation via thought therapy to

- ultimately create a state of relaxation,
- enable the subconscious to speak easier to the still mind,
- allow feelings to be heard and memories explored and rationalised, therefore transforming into positivity.

Sounds like a good thing? Energy flows through the meridian lines – the energy channels between the chakras increase when one is relaxed and in a state of flow. We are more able to 'hear' divine wisdom when the mind is still, the heart is open and receptive, and we have requested/allowed the ego, the conscious mind, to have a rest. When we invite, allow, acknowledge, and act according to divine inspiration, good things happen. Synchronicity appears to be the norm. Things just turn out, and we know what we need to do.

As described in <u>Science of Happiness</u> one can see again the similarity between the various messages being promoted through millennia. In summary, the seven habits of happiness are as follows:

- In relationships, express your heart to those who are close and important to you.

- Perform acts of kindness and help and support others where they are at.

- Exercise and look after yourself by moving and eating well. Both lifts the mood and keeps the body strong, moves body fluids, and removes wastes.

- Work within the space that are suited to your skills and with which we experience joy or passion.

- Spiritual engagement and meaning connects you to something greater than ourselves that is not another human – nature, the universe, or divine with which you communicate through your highest self and 'knowing'.

- Strengths and virtues, are one's own talents and unique strengths. Use them to your advantage in the now, and use them for the greater good, and not only one's own.

- Having a positive mindset means being grateful and thankful from your heart, feeling the emotion and allowing it to be for all that one is and does.

I ask you, how different are these premises from other religions, spiritual practices, etc.?

Self-actualisation or attainment doesn't happen all at once. It can be a slow, stepping-stone process. It may seem that steps taken forward are quickly stepped back as different situations 'press your buttons'. Each time something comes up, you are being given the opportunity to check if the belief or value is still important to keep, to alter, or to get rid of. This is the beauty and the purpose of it all. From a Godly religious point of view, it is to ask ourselves, 'What would love do now?' From Eastern philosophy, it is 'What is the correct thing to do?' After coming from a place of peace, love, and humility.

It takes time, and just as 'school' repeatedly goes over the material in class, homework, and assignments, life too gives us repeated opportunities to experience ourselves to see who we are in the moment and the opportunity for change. Again, each time we come across the same scenarios, we are being put to the test of clarity, strengthening our belief of what we choose to stand for and how!

As we gain more insight, wisdom, and compassion and as we work from love and not ego, our filters, beliefs, values, and vows start to change. It gets easier to work from a space of love and compassion, simply because the filter is getting cleaner and not as clogged up on the limiting beliefs and blocks we previously placed there.

We Operate from Either Love or Fear

Ultimately, we operate either out of fear (or unloving) or out of love, and as in the world of business, it is important to work with mentors whom you want to become more like. With their help and gentle probing, you can quickly see which of these two sides, love or fear, you are currently operating from. Your mentor, healer, or counsellor can then help you to move towards a more loving and supportive concept of self, which will influence all situations around you as you live from a space of love and truth. There are many different modalities to help you determine the 'issues' and help reverse the impact on your life. It is invaluable to access the subconscious mind and 'rewrite'.

As you can imagine, fear or its cousin, low self-esteem, which stems from the fear of not being lovable, creates the negatives in life. It is contracting and the subconscious will create safe or known situations to ensure you, as a person, are safe. It works within the lower chakra. This is in line with Maslow's belief about security: feeling safe within your environment; ability to earn or create sufficient money to provide the basic necessities of life – food, clothing, shelter, and medical treatment; ability to stand up for yourself and your beliefs as you see them; feeling good at home; and social and familial law and order. This isn't about facing the fear through action only but by addressing the reason for the fear in the first place.

The first step, as in any program, is awareness – what is going on at the moment, how do you feel about it, and what or how would you like things to be different? From the answers to these questions, you can start making conscious choices of what beliefs, thoughts, and actions to keep, change, or throw out. It is also a good starting place to gain insight into whom you may need assistance from.

Making a conscious decision to change means taking personal responsibility for your own thoughts that have created your circumstances, your current situation, and your health. Once you take this responsibility, it is yours to direct your life in the manner in which you choose. A commitment to yourself is vital. Mine, over time, developed into 'to operate from a place of truth and love'.

- 'To operate from my values, and not from others, with giving myself the opportunity to clarify what is mine or others' belief, interpretation, should, expectation.'

> 'Own my part of the problems that I see and work towards understanding why I see them as problems, where the thoughts come from and what can I do to encourage a win-win solution.'

It is so useful to get to the underlying reason as to why things are the way they are, and then if you choose, release the negative hold they have over your life. You might need help with this part as the entanglement of emotions, the energy hooks that keep them attached to our being, and energy can be phenomenal. I suggest considering a number of possible energy healing methods, such as meditation, hypnosis, reiki, kinesiology, bars, or any that you are drawn to do. You may find that one style of change works better with one issue, or a series of issues, or even the level of change you are at. Just like you wouldn't send an infant to a university lecture to learn about the chemistry of baby food and expect them to 'get it', respect the level of change you are at and match it best to that level. You may even find that some issues need a university level of insight, and others will be just on faith. It is what you need at the moment, just as infants trust their parents to look after them in the right way. Above all, and this is paramount, ask around, and speak with practitioners before you delve into a method. Test the water, so to speak, and be sure you feel OK and safe. If you feel safe with the person and the modality, shifts are easier to create. Remember too that a different person or modality may be required for different issues or stage of life.

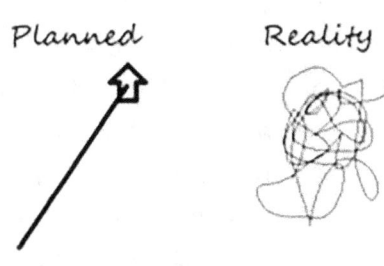

It is one thing to have therapy, but you also need to apply and practice it. Just like all other skills, change or growth, regular reflection of how you were before and after therapy. Making very aware choices and noticing the subtleness of life makes it easier and faster.

> Don't panic if things seem to take time or you are going around in circles. Going back to the illustration of change reality, it can be messy and all over the place. All that matters at the end of the day is your intention to progress, that you are putting the effort in, and you are acknowledging with gratitude for the smallest of things. Ground yourself and reward yourself with nature, pets, children, love, and friendships that support you. There is little point hanging out with friends or partners who are demoralising, diminishing, or unsupportive. If you are in an abusive or risky situation, then seek help. You are worth so much more than being emotionally, physical, mentally, or spiritually abused. Others have made change, so can you. Not easy, but possible. If you prefer to keep change within the psychological and emotional framework, then the following steps towards a more positive mental attitude may be helpful.

Mindfulness Activity

There are several steps to changing your thoughts and adopting a more positive mental attitude.

- ➢ Become an optimist.

- ➢ Become aware of self-talk.

- ➢ Ask better questions.

- Employ positive affirmations.
- Set positive goals.
- Practice positive visualisations.
- Laugh long and often.
- Read or listen to inspiring messages.

Thank goodness for Facebook, Pinterest, and Instagram because we can now keep notes of our inspired moments and affirmations.

Step 1: Learn optimism.

Pessimists tend to see the world in a heavy or negative way. It is worth learning how to be optimistic. Studies have shown that optimists are healthier and happier. They enjoy life more; they tend to have deeper, loving friendships. Learning optimism means getting into the habit of seeing the world in a more positive light. If you are pessimistic, that is OK. It is only because you formed the habit of negative thinking. Since you have learnt it, it means you can unlearn it.

If you wish to assess how you see the world or cope with situations from a mind level check out the Authentic Happiness website and complete some of the questionnaires. The questionnaires may help you understand yourself, how you perceive the world around you and how you respond to it.

The remaining steps can help condition your attitude to become positive.

Step 2: Become aware of self-talk.

We all talk to ourselves, all the time. There is a constant dialogue going on in our heads, what we feel and think; our opinions on things, people, and conversations; and what we think and feel about ourselves. Our self-talk operates from our subconscious mind's filter and reinforces our perception or point of view onto our conscious mind. To develop or maintain a positive mental attitude, it is invaluable to note when negative thoughts creep in and work towards changing that point of view. Play the flip game - seeing the situation from the opposite side and see if there is a possibility of shifting a bit towards that standpoint.

Guard yourself against negative self-talk, become aware of your common threads of self-talk, and then consciously work towards imprinting positive messages on your subconscious mind. Take more notice of nature. Even five minutes looking at the wonder of nature or babies can be enough to start melting a heavy or upset mind. Two powerful tools in creating positive self-talk are questions and affirmations. Complete the exercise <u>Self-Talk, Self-Awareness</u> to gain extra clarity of who is 'talking' to you. The talk gently exercise discussed earlier can also help forgive and let go.

Step 3: Ask better questions.

Questions are one of the most powerful ways to make a difference in your life. When we ask questions with the intent to understand, we can appreciate why people do, say, and behave in the ways they do. It develops insight which can lead to compassion, a very healing emotion.

When we apply questions to ourselves, with compassion, we have the opportunity to review our actions, thoughts, and beliefs that have controlled our life to date. Again, when applied with curiosity and not judgement, we can see why and how we took on other people's ideals. The quality of self-talk and therefore the quality of our lives is influenced by the answers to quality questions.

To get to the root issues about our life and in particular the things we don't like, questions asked in a specific manner can probe into the subconscious. This is well documented by Anthony Robbins and many others. These questions are fundamental tools for change. According to Robbins in <u>Awaken the Giant Within</u>, the quality of your life is equal to the quality of the questions you habitually ask yourself. He teaches that whatever question you ask your brain, it will answer. While there are many other people who have excelled in this field, <u>Brendon Burchard</u> has written several excellent books (in my view anyway) that describe mind change, methods, and stories to facilitate change in the rational mind.

Regardless of the situation, asking better questions is bound to clarify your true belief system so you can improve your attitude. Better questions pave the way through problem solving and thinking outside the square to some really unique solutions. If you want to have a better life, simply ask better questions. It sounds simple because it is. If you want more energy, excitement, and/or happiness in your life, simply ask yourself the following questions on a consistent basis.

Give these a whirl.

> *What am I most happy about in my life right now?*
> *Why does that make me happy?*
> *How does that make me feel?*
>
> *What am I most excited about in my life right now?*
> *Why does that make me excited?*
> *How does that make me feel?*
>
> *What am I most grateful about in my life right now?*

Why does that make me grateful?
How does that make me feel?

What am I enjoying most in my life right now?
What about that do I enjoy?
How does that make me feel?

What am I committed to in my life right now?
Why am I committed to that?
How does that make me feel?

Who do I love? (Starting close and moving out)
Who loves me?
What must I do today to achieve my long-term goal?

When the student is ready, the teacher appears. Likewise, when the teacher is ready, the students appear. Which are you?

When you are searching for answers to life's challenges, and ask these types of questions, you will be drawn to the best teachers, solutions, partnerships, experiences, etc., to help create the answers.

You have an opportunity to transform limited beliefs and programs into positive messages or, better still, let them go and transform them into light. Reprogramming your subconscious into believing that you have an abundant, healthy, love-filled life or the opposite of what you're experiencing does the work; and your subconscious mind, with your spirit, can begin to create it.

Another avenue to assessing the subconscious beliefs and the impact they have on your life is through kinesiology, which is a process where questions asked are directed to the individual but are answered by body responses. It is an interesting area and worthwhile considering to help yourself understand the underlying reasons for why you have created your current life and body. Reprogramming reverses the beliefs or limiting thoughts that are holding you back in life. The journey meditation work combines all these methods into a single process. For an effective change and clearing effect, consider this type of work.

Step 4: Employ positive affirmations.

An affirmation is a statement made with emotional intensity. Just as negative statements leave an imprint on the subconscious mind, so do the positive affirmations to create healthy, positive self-images. Affirmations support the desired changes you declare on the premise the subconscious doesn't know if what is being said is real or not. Therefore, we can 'fake it until you make it'.

Louise Hay is one pioneer in the area of creating life changes. The relationships between thoughts and medical diseases are accurately described in her book You Can Heal Your Life. Hay also includes an entire section on positive affirmations to support the subconscious mind in making positive changes to the body's health and healing.

The way to make affirmations the most effective is to think about the mental cause of the situation and analyse how it could be your pattern or programming that has attracted the situation to mirror your belief. Ask yourself, 'What are the thoughts in me that have created this?' Continue asking quality questions until you feel confident you know the root cause of the situation. Use *Opposite Hand Writing* technique spoken about already then say to yourself:

"I am willing to release the pattern in my subconscious that has created this condition."

> I am willing to release the pattern in my subconscious that has created this condition.

Explore the silver lining of the experience – what are the good parts of what is happening, then go create the affirmation that focuses on the silver lining and what you aim to create change, choose to have more of, or work towards.

Repeat the affirmation to yourself several times, preferably out loud or in front of a mirror. Assume that healing of your thoughts and body has commenced, and then continue. Repeat the affirmation each time the situation is thought of.

Some useful affirmations to start making the changes could include the following:

> *I am blessed with an abundance of energy!*
>
> *Love, joy, and happiness flow through me with every heartbeat. I am thankful to God for all of my good fortune.*
>
> *YES, I CAN!*

An experience I have often had is when the thought 'Money seems tight' comes up, I sit and reflect on what is here. When I go to the space of wonder, acknowledgement, and gratitude, it is easy to see I really do feel I have the perfect life. I have freedom to choose what I do; I have a home, in the perfect spot for me; and I am getting back to what I love. Money is sufficient, and when I work from the space of wow and thanks, money really does seem to pop into my bank account. It can be from people who owe me money or a discount or a surprise, but it is enough to pay for what I need, and then some. I have experienced this time and again. When the chips were down, the money angels would visit. The more I saw them, the more they turned up to bless me.

Louise has an entire affirmations book *Heart Thoughts*, which highlights on almost every aspect of life. This may be worth investing in to support you during change and to create a positive space from which you can draw strength.

Simple affirmations guidelines.

It is important to have fun with them! If you are struggling to create a positive affirmation because of negative self-talk or resistance to creating a positive affirmation on a point, the resistance is bringing your attention to an issue that would be best addressed with clearing/ processing work. Tap it out and/or complete the forgiveness exercise. Allow the feelings to transform into a much lighter version and let yourself be freer to get on with what you love to be and do.

Generally, positive affirmations can help make you feel really good

if you follow these guidelines.

Always phrase an affirmation in the present tense.

Imagine that it has already come to pass.

Always phrase the affirmation as a positive statement.

Avoid using the words 'not' and 'never'.

Do your best to totally associate with the positive feeling that is generated by the affirmation.

Create a movie packed with as many sensations as possible. At first you might find it challenging to 'know' how it feels the feeling you want to have associated with the statements. I can only suggest watching movies and getting a sense of what the feelings are and then replicating these in the movie statement.

Keep the affirmation short and simple, but full of feeling. Be creative.

The affirmation doesn't have long or complicated, it is about affirming the 'point' of the affirmation

Imagine yourself really experiencing what you are affirming.

Create the end product movie showing you walking around and doing what you are affirming.

For instance, let's work with the affirmation I am performing the job of my choice. This for myself is writing. I love the process of getting my ideas gleaned from other's research and presentations and putting it into everyday operation. I also love reading. So, my movie goes something like this.

I see myself at the computer in a space that is aspiring and comfortable. I see the words being written on the computer screen, and I feel excited, enthusiastic, buzzing with excitement as I see the transformation happening. I then move forward to seeing the material being read by others, on their computer, in books that look absolutely fabulous with their covers, their colour, and the feel of the book in their hands. The reader is experiencing 'ahhhh' moments of comprehension. They are making choices and working out how they need to make changes that suit them.

The next scene is me presenting the material onstage, and people love the way I present, relate, and talk with them. They get that I have struggled and crawled with fingernails at times to get to where I am at the time, just like they have too. The feeling at this stage is awe and gratitude, amazement, wonder at how amazing I am (not in a crazy way) but acknowledging myself as I would another who has gone through similar experiences. I then have the blessing of coming back to my space and sitting in the space of thankfulness, gratitude, and awe that I had it in me to begin with and that I had the courage to allow it out.

We all have greatness in us, but it is our own perceived limitations that keep us small, just as Marianne Williamson wrote about earlier in her speech on being small. How about you, what do visualise when you give yourself permission to dream however small or big it is for you?

Make the affirmation personal to you and full of meaning.

Using these guidelines and examples, write down five affirmations that apply to you. Write out what it is you are grateful for and what it is you are working towards creating. State these affirmations aloud while you are taking your shower, driving, or doing daily chores.

Pretty much all business development books focus on mindset or frame of mind for business success. If it works in the business world to create goals, change beliefs and one's perception at the thinking level, then it will work in any other area of your life. It is also in line with the principles of the law of attraction advocated by Norman Vincent Peale and Dale Carnegie in the early parts of the last century.

The universal law of what you focus on you attract is also written in the Bible: 'Seek and you shall find. Ask and you will receive.' Naturally, there is a bit more to it, but the premise is still there.

Be careful what you wish for, the amount of time you focus on something, and be sure you are super clear as to what you are putting out there. The subconscious doesn't know what is real or fiction. It only sees, feels, and knows what you are projecting onto its field of operation. 'OK, this is what she/he is asking for – oh, it has a lot of attention to detail and has lots of emotion in it. Better give it in spades. It is what they are really concentrating on.' From my own experience, it is true what you focus on is what you get, even the really, really bad stuff, and who could I 'blame'? Me for worrying about things that I couldn't influence and not looking at the brighter side of the situation and what I have and what I am asking for more good stuff in.

Step 5: Set positive goals.

Setting goals in a way that results in a positive experience is another powerful method to build a positive attitude and raise self-esteem. Goals can be used to create a success cycle. Achieving goals helps you feel better about yourself, and the better you feel about yourself, the more likely you are to achieve your goals.

Here are some guidelines to use when setting goals:

Start with small, practical, and achievable goals. Too big and even the critical self in the subconscious will laugh and sabotage your endeavours.

- State the goal in positive terms; do not use any negative words in your goal statement. For example, it is better to say, 'I enjoy eating healthy, low kJ, nutritious foods' than 'I will not eat sugar, candy, ice cream, and other fattening foods.' The mind will hear sugar, ice cream, and fattening food and start looking for it.

- Make your goal attainable and realistic. For example, if you are fully grown and five feet tall, it isn't very realistic to set the goal of becoming a professional basketball player with the height of six feet.

If you are not used to setting goals, start out with ones that are easily attainable. Like getting up in the mornings at a specific time or being punctual. Again, goals can be used to create a success cycle and a positive self-image. Little things add up to make a major difference in the way you feel about yourself. Explore the work of Keith Abraham, he is a goal and passion coach. You can find him at keithabraham.com

When you have success, follow through with healthier step, healthier goals towards bigger, bolder goals, and more out there. The subconscious, and the view you hold about yourself, is powerful, and I am suggesting healing yourself so the ride is easier and less fraught with angst. Mind the harder you push, the quicker your 'stuff' will rise to be looked at, cleared, and healed.

- *Be specific, in line with the affirmation. The more clarity there is, in detail with the emotion, the more likely you are to reach it.* For example, if you want to become healthier, what type of health do you desire? What changes do you want to make to achieve this? Clearly define what it is you want to achieve. Create the scenario you would like your body to create. Which organ system do you require to be involved? What is it, or what are they doing to correct the issue? What is the emotional trigger? What is the trade-off that the body has figured out and chosen to support? (This is another topic for another book.)

- State the goal in the present tense, not the future tense. To reach your goal, you have to believe that you have already attained it. You must literally program yourself to have achieved the goal. See and feel yourself having already achieved the goal and success will be yours.

- Make them passionate, because the more you feel, believe, and taste it, the more you are likely to strive for it. It will have meaning and reason in it even if no one else 'gets it'!

- Create a story outlining all the good parts of the experience you are working towards. Include lots of descriptive words describing what your life, your typical day, activities etc. What does it look and feel? What are the things you are doing with yourself, your family, your special someone? How is your career going? What targets have you already achieved? The more details with as many positive descriptive words, the better. Read it, feel it, and see it as many times a day as possible. Remember, the subconscious mind doesn't know if it is a memory, a story, or reality, so you might as well maximise the opportunity to create what you are desirous of. If it isn't in your best interest because there are still things that need to be learnt or transformed or others are not quite ready, then your desires may take longer to manifest. Don't give up; commit to the creation, transformation, release, and growth.

Now let's write at least one affirmation together.

I want to have a better life, more love, peace, and joy. This could be written as...

I am now experiencing a fully vibrant life, filled with love, peace, and joy.

What is the thing you would like to change?

_____

How do you want it to be?

_____

_____

Now word it in the positive...

I (your name) or I (your name); It is now

_____

_____

Here are eight tips to help you have more laughter in your life:

1. Learn to laugh at yourself. Recognise how funny some of your behaviours really are. We all have quirkiness or behaviours that are ours and ours alone that are truly funny and don't need to be taken seriously.

2. Add humour into activities if appropriate. People love to laugh. Get a joke book to learn how to tell a good joke. Laughter is life's medicine, so why not make life enjoyable?

3. Read comics. Find one that's funny and follow it. Humour is very individual. What I may find funny, you may not.

4. Watch comedies on TV or DVDs.

5. Go to the movies with a friend. Generally, you will feed off each other's laughter during and after the movie. Not only do you share the joy, it will help build strong relationships.

6. Listen to comedy tapes while driving.

7. Play with kids. Kids really know how to laugh and play. If you do not have kids of your own, spend time with nieces, nephews, or neighborhood children. Become a big brother or sister. Investigate little athletics, or volunteer at organisations where kids are.

8. Ask yourself, 'What is funny about this?' Why wait till later to look back on the funny side of life? Take the time to see the funny side right now. Not only will it help to break the tension, it may well open up the mind to recognising workable solutions. Find the humor in the situation and enjoy a good laugh immediately.

One Step at a Time

Remember, any voyage begins with one step and is followed by many other steps. Remember to set short-term goals that can be used to help you achieve your long-term goals. Get into the habit of asking yourself the following question each morning and evening:

What must I do today to achieve my long-term goal?

As Mike Litman of Connect to Success, Inc., has so plainly put it, 'Ask yourself: what are two small steps I can take right now that can move me forward?

Then do it NOW!'

It is important to understand at this point that as movement or change towards your desired outcome begins, all sorts of things may happen. The sensation of two steps forward and one step back is very possible. Why? Because the mind is preserving 'known' behaviours and beliefs, making changes, allowing other unlocked beliefs to surface. This is the time to trial and strengthen new beliefs you are changing. Basically, the mind is attempting to do two things – keep things as they are known within its comfort zone and help you address hidden fears and negative beliefs and to help you become clear by asking the conscious mind, 'Is this is what you want?' It is vital, during any process of growth or change, to be very aware of your own thoughts. Hidden treasures will arise. How you investigate and handle them will determine your outcome.

Sabotage

Sabotage is a common, almost natural response to change. It is the mind's way of resisting change and maintaining its known position. Sabotage is easiest to see when things are moving forward. It is a self-protection mechanism designed to keep you safe, because somewhere in your past you have made an association 'that this = that and from here on, I (the subconscious) must ensure it doesn't happen again'. You might be choosing healthier foods when suddenly a locked-in belief or feeling about a similar event (previous attempt, or the hidden belief that you don't deserve to be lighter and beautiful) is released during the change. WHAM! Sabotage stops you in your tracks, does the opposite to what you have chosen to do, and makes you feel not so good about yourself.

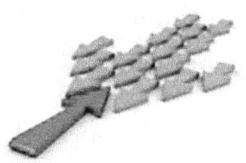

Sabotage has the potential to stop or negate any further progress. Sabotage is a very common and powerful tool the subconscious mind uses to protect us from the unknown. One way to move through sabotages is to explore any negative thought, feeling, sensation, change in the body, or relationship. Explore the key issue or feeling that are rising up, allow these feelings, and aha moments etc give you insight into what is really going on. Ask quality questions and organise some process work to help unlock the core and release the block so you can continue to move forward, just like taking away a bottom card of pyramid causes the entire concept to fall. Childhood memories, school situations, previous relationships, messages of being unloved, unworthy, inadequate, etc., will, if not looked at with a loving hand, negate any progress being made. Change is an ongoing journey.

There are four steps to changing:

1. Monitor your progress towards your desired outcome. Become aware of things you are doing to achieve this goal.

2. When things become harder, or you are tempted to do something different from the 'plan', work through them. Ask direct questions in relation to the goal and path you are working towards. Be truthful of the answers; listen to the first response that comes to mind. This is often the most truthful.

3. Ask yourself if the answer is a truth or a belief that supports your goal or plan. If it is a belief you would like to keep within your belief system, keep it. Otherwise, do process work to place the belief in the positive. Whatever the answer, it is OK, because this is your life and journey, and things will be different when you are ready for change.

4. If you choose to change the belief the mind gave you to the questions, it is a matter of rewriting the script to the positive opposite of the one given.

The more beliefs or issues looked at, the more aware you become that your feelings are creating your circumstances. You gain greater power to create change. You reclaim your ability to recreate a better you as described by the values, beliefs, and desires you would like your life to be.

One way to do this is to sit quietly and ask,

'What is influencing the negative feeling/ thought/ situation / illness / disease?'

'What in my past is trapped and attempting to be looked at to make a difference now?'

'What do I need to know, feel, or do to change it?'

Step 6: Practice positive visualisations.

Positive visualisation or imagery is another powerful tool in creating health, happiness, or success. Two other excellent books to support your making subconscious changes are *The Inner Edge* and *Living in Balance*. Both present ways to see our lives the way we want them to be before it happens. Mindvalley.com and Hayhouse.com are two other fantastic sources for a whole range of self-help methods ranging from meditations, theory, and affirmations to clearing and releasing work.

If you wish to work on it yourself, picture yourself in ideal health if you truly want to experience this state. You can use visualisation in all areas of your life, but especially in your health. In fact, some of the most promising research on the power of visualisation involves improving the immune system to reverse the health issue. Be creative and have fun with positive visualisations and you will soon find yourself living your dreams. It is our dreams that propel us as we roll through this life. They are powerful and inspirational. In fact, the famous author Anatole France said something about dreams and life that really hits home.

In the topic of describing or creating dreams, Stephen Covey in *The Seven Habits of Highly Effective People* suggests a very powerful technique – to write in as much detail as possible what you would like people to say about you when you died. What characteristics would you like to be remembered for? Who would remember you the most fondly, and for what, your family, children, friends, acquaintances, work colleagues, etc.? Are there charitable funds you would like to be associated with? What activities will you be remembered for? This technique in essence helps you to define in detail your life's mission statement, something that you can be accountable for and use as a yardstick when things seem to be going off course. It will help you design your life, from which the everyday actions are made from.

Another is to describe again, in as much detail, your perfect day. What would you wear, where would you be, who would you be with, and what would you do? Which friends would you be with? Would you like to give a speech? If so, what would you say? What characteristics would you like to show or exemplify during this time?

This technique can be used in all aspects of your life. Look at your life wheel. Is it in balance? How is it matching to your eulogy ideal? What areas still need modification to create balance and a smoother life ride?

Step 7: Laugh long and often.

By laughing frequently and taking a lighter view of life, you will find that life is much more enjoyable and fun. Researchers are discovering that laughter enhances the immune system and promotes improved physiology. Recent medical research has also confirmed that laughter enhances the blood flow to the body's extremities and improves cardiovascular function. It plays an active part in the body's release of endorphins and other natural mood-elevating and painkilling chemicals and improves the transfer of oxygen and nutrients to internal organs.

Summary

So, there you go, something to ponder I hope. I also hope that you were able to glean even a small amount of insight and inspiration from what you have just read. This is only a snowflake of information on top of an iceberg. There is so much more information available on these very thoughts.

Change is a desired state if one is working towards self-fulfilment or to be the best one can be at any given moment. It leads us to become quite clear as to who we are at the time and gives us an opportunity to modify this to be more in line with our preferred way of being. We are given the opportunity to create something we would like to be. The concept has been around since the beginning of time and in every culture to date. Each has aspired to extend their knowledge, skills, and, for some more than others, power. Core religious and spiritual teachings inspire the same principles, and love is the highest possible vibration or tenant, to which we mortals are to aspire towards by laying down our humanness and taking up more of divinity/spirit/universal love to fill the void created in the wake of 'letting go'.

Physical and emotional discord is seen as the flow of energy and selflove is either being blocked or being channelled around the blocked areas in the body. This disruption in flow alters physical and chemical functions, which in turn creates symptoms. The closer we look at the symptoms for their hidden messages, and not only in pathology, physical alignment, or symptom control, the faster our body can heal and continue on its journey to fulfilment or self-actualisation.

Fortunately, we are living in an era of change. Many are becoming aware of these very topics, and consumer dis-satisfaction with the medical paradigm is transforming awareness into a more holistic approach to life. People are starting to take more care of themselves with body care – massages, yoga, mindfulness and meditation, and exercise; food choices are moving away from convenience foods towards whole, organic where possible. As a community, we are becoming less tolerant of harmful behaviours against others, with the rise of calling out on crimes against women and children and abuse of power. We are encouraging one another to be more tolerant, accepting, supportive, and compassionate, to reach out and help one another and not push other people down.

I think we are on the verge of a collective breakthrough rising to another level of living. Countries that have their foundational needs in place are using their hearts and voices to give and protect those countries who are being victimised. We are organising mass meditations and consciousness-raising activities, which, when organised within a group setting, multiply the intensity of the focus.

Change starts within ourselves! It is up to us to see where we are at, see where or what we would rather be, and then take steps to evolve into our preferred state. It is not up to the government, our parents, our teachers, our employers, etc. Their role is to put things in place to stimulate productivity and clarity. Ultimately, it is us that make the difference. We are the ones who choose how to respond to the environments and situations we find ourselves in. It is up to us to learn the skills and strengthen them so we can be the best we possibly can be. It is up to us to work towards our actualisation and support others along the way to be the best they can be, for if we evolve together, then, as a community, nation, and country and humanity, we are creating a much healthier place to be in.

To have personalized support to transform and heal from your limiting beliefs and create the life you want explore www.stepstochange.com.au.

About the Author

Leah is a medically trained dietitian, who understands the Medical Model of care, but also felt that had to be another way of healing. Inner healing towards health is her passion and her desire to make a difference in your life. With her own personal experience of severe depression, gut issues, inexplainable, severe neck pain through her adolescence Leah, knows and understands. Challenging life events further triggered migraines, lower back pain and ongoing stress refocused her passion to understanding what, how and why her body was 'falling apart'.

Leah realised different questions needed to be asked and her quest took her on many different healing paths, all led by personal challenges, her food sensitivity reactions and desire for deep healing. The need to understand how natural occurring chemicals alter body chemistry, can alter moods, trigger memories, activate gene expression and create a wide variety of 'undiagnosable' symptoms made the quest even more intriguing.

Following her life path of healing her body, mind and soul Leah is part of the deep holistic movement that encourages individuals to explore their own soul needs by supporting you to learn your own body language that is being spoken through your symptoms triggered by foods enabling you to reclaim your balance and inner you. You deserve to be nourished, loved and treated with reverence. Feed your soul, feed your body and allow yourself to come back to you.

About the Book

This book is a broad introduction how everything we do, think, feel, and are exposed to changes our body chemistry and ultimately our body and mind. Our body is a combination of compounds and just as in the science beaker when different compounds, temperature, or pressure changes our body changes in response.

Our individual reactions are unique based on our genes, life experiences and what one has internalised. Our body symptoms, and life constantly give us clues, asking us to look into our self-perceptions, so we come back to the most important thing – love. How? By learning the language of our body symptoms, transforming heavy emotions into light and love, unlocking the hidden treasure – your truest self. This is our duty. Are you up to the challenge?

www.ingramcontent.com/pod-product-compliance
Lightning Source LLC
Chambersburg PA
CBHW052104070526
44584CB00017B/2336